GUIDE TO INTERMITTENT FASTING

Reset metabolism, Lose Weight Without a Diet and Heal Your Health Through Fasting Methods 16:8, 5:2 And Eat-Stop-Eat!

- Author –

Linda D. Parker

Codice ISBN: 9781688443334

TABLE OF CONTENTS

Foreword

This book titled *"Guide to Intermittent Fasting"* is written to escalate the basics of intermittent fasting and various methods to accomplish these fasting situations, and their implications for humans, together with their pros and cons for the human body. These involve various researches, pre-carious plot and easy to understand writings. It is actually authored by keeping in mind the writer's caliber and belongingness. Therefore, one who reads this will let himself taking over the world of actualities and relatedness. One who is looking for the methods to cater to the over-weight issues must read this material and will love it due to its comprehensiveness, preparedness, and benefits to them, without demanding much. These best part about it is no specific demand for intermittent fasting as it doesn't need to skip delicious foods or food of own choice. It just restricts calorie intake for some time to mend your body into a sound and healthy one. Being a writer, I am sure that the reader will love it and will act according to it to gain more benefits and favorable outcomes.

INTRODUCTION

Why you should read this book?

Aperson who is worried of his raised weight or accumulated fats to turn his body into a chubby one, must not waste his time in finding dieting ways that are hectic and tough to try on and caters less benefit and more harm. He must switch to a more rational way that is, in fact, the way of Intermittent Fasting. This method is centuries long tested and recommended by every single religious scholar or a nutritional expert and doctor.

Intermittent fasting involves methods according to your needs and requirements and implications are too easy that can be adopted by a child too. If you wanna try intermittent fasting, you must read this book. This book provides you an opportunity of all and sundry about intermittent fasting and will let you aware of all the types, their requisitions, implications, food to opt and foods to avoid and work out best for you according to the method opted. Thus, in detail, each and everything about intermittent fasting now becomes accessible through this book, which entails all in all about intermittent fasting. Therefore, it is a must-read the book and acknowledge your attention and steer you to the right path together with its implications and benefits accumulated together at one point.

This book if tried and tested with various methods of intermittent fasting and twisted around with methods could find a viable way for them to rely on intermittent fasting and let them acquire their benefits with less effort and high gain ratio.

The compelling attitude and approach of the topic

This topic is purely a delight for those who are looking to divert their thinking towards rational behavior on weight loss and reshaping body parts or muscles to gain safe and sound shape of the body. People love to seek benefit with less effort and fewer findings to gain more on account of fasting. Intermittent fasting is not a fad or a craze dreamt up without basis in fact, but a regime that is founded on hard science.

The purpose of the following chapter is to present and summarize the scientific literature that is available regarding the benefits of intermittent fasting and to allow you to draw your own conclusions. I feel strongly that it is important for you to be satisfied with the science and convinced by the data before you begin your own race.

A comparable proportion of people who are willing to give their suggestions on a program of intermittent fasting courageously do so in order to achieve a reduction in body weight. And, this is a perfectly tangible goal in its own right. However, you will find out more as you progress with your regime that a number of other health benefits become wide open and disclosed. For example, you may find that you have more energy, that you suffer fewer coughs and colds, and that you feel generally in a better state of health. There are a number of further advantages to this program which may not be immediately noticeable but which will improve your underlying health in general. For example, data show that intermittent fasting has positive effects in terms of cardiovascular health, neurological function, protection against disease, insulin sensitivity, and hormonal responses. The scientific evidence to support the benefits of intermittent fasting in these different areas is discussed in the following chapters.

CHAPTER 1

Intermittent Fasting and Its Implications to Human Body

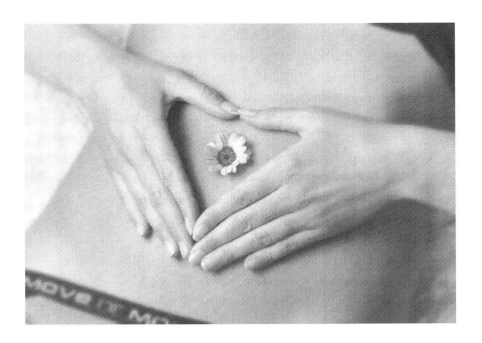

Fasting is a way of self-control or restraint from physical or body-related activities or food ingestion of each and every type that is according to some will and could benefit the body by losing surplus fat and growing the body muscles to ideality. The perfect way out is to leave one or more meals for some time, drawn on the basis of your stamina. This stamina is built by practicing more and more. The fasting either did for religious purpose or for physical purposes, could benefit and shape the body by losing weight, surplus fat and irregularities. Fasting has many implications and types according to its formations and timespan. Here the under-consideration type is Intermittent Fasting. Let's move to this type.

1.1. What is intermittent fasting?

A lot of fasting methods and techniques discussed across the globe and tested to signify their strengths and weaknesses but the results vary at large and show irregular flow and arbitrary trends. The most significant method extracted out and tested viciously is Intermittent Fasting. This is one of the most popular methods of fasting across the globe and formulates the eating patterns based on derivations of timeframe and calorie consumption. This way of fasting involves alternating eating and fasting cycles that allows one to formulate eating patterns and develop eating habits according to the calorie consumption and fat dissolving. The researches have suggested that this way of fasting involves causes and implications that contribute to weight loss, health appraisal, improved metabolic health, immunity building against diseases, and contributing to live a healthier life. The more approach oriented it is, the more vicious results come out.

Intermittent fasting is a class of fasting where one switch between the periods of fasting and eating and allows his/her body to settle down between these cycles. It doesn't involve the type of food to eat. It involves the pattern to eat and timeframe when to eat. More elaborately, this is a way of scheduling your meals to get the most out of them and get a lot by consuming less. Therefore, one can assume it is not a technique which involves what to eat. It is rather a technique that involves when to eat. This is not a diet in a conventional sense. It is a pattern of when to eat. There are several different methods to elaborate intermittent fasting. All of which involves splitting of a day or a week into eating patterns suitable to your stamina perceptions. People across the globe use fasting as a technique to follow on a daily basis whenever they sleep. This method if applied for a little longer time frame could be termed as intermittent fasting.

A simpler approach to this one is skipping breakfast and eating your first meal of the day at lunch and eating dinner at night. Just skipping your breakfast in the morning and making it your habit to ingest fewer calories could be a better approach to intermittent fasting. In this way, you are actually fasting for around 16 hours in a whole day from dinner at night to lunch at noon on the very next day. This is one of the popular fasting ways of intermittent fasting and is known as the 16/8 approach.

Talking about the evolutionary history of the man, fasting has always been a practice in the past. There are traces of fasting in every era in the past and now it also serves as an obligation somewhere and exercise or tonic somewhere else. In the past, when there were no refrigerators, and no preservations, food couldn't be stored at long. Therefore, it was consumed as a whole and after that, some days might come, when there was no food, no prey then humans go on without eating at a longer span of time and fasting is exercised. The body get used to it after continuous attempts of fasting and develops a habit of fasting.

It is pretty much natural to go for fasting as our bodies are adaptive to fasting and formulated to cater up to the fasting needs. Each and every process of the body start re-structuring and re-organization with continuous fasting. Whenever we fast, our bodies start to reduce blood sugar, stimulates insulin production, and production of human growth hormone is increased drastically. This approach of fasting come up with various benefits such as weight loss, stimulating metabolic health, burning fats and helping to live longer. It also helps in building protection against diseases like heart diseases, diabetes, and Alzheimer disease, etc. Therefore, it is termed as a simpler life hack that will make your life simple, while enhancing the hormone growth and reducing the fats and make your body muscular.

Let's move towards understanding the phenomenon of intermittent fasting that how it works well for a body. We will first understand the phenomenon of fat loss by differentiating between the fed state and the fasted state. When you are eating and digesting food, your body is in the fed state. This stage starts when you start eating and lasts long 4 to 5 hours after eating as this time involves digesting the food. In this state, a very hard thing for the body is to burn already stored fat because the insulin levels are high in the body. This is the fed state.

Afterward, the next stage comes, when you are not digesting the food and your body is done with digesting the already ate meal. In this stage, your body starts to burn already stored fat as insulin levels are low. This stage lasts as long as 8 to 12 hours after eating a meal. Your body starts reaching the fat that was inaccessible during the fed state. If we continuously go on to indulge in this fasted state, our bodies will develop the habit of burning already stored fat and as a result, we will start losing weight. Indulging in the intermittent fasting state isn't require especially what you eat, how much you eat, and how often you exercise, etc.

Let's move towards the effects of bodily processes of intermittent fasting.

1.2. How it affects your Cells and Hormones?

Fasting is a way to regularize your body's functions and re-organize the structuring of the body that is affected due to fat production. Fasting directly impacts fats and hormone production. Whenever you fast, several things start happening in your body at the cellular and molecular level. Hormonal growth and hormone production is stimulated according to the needs of the body and to make them idealized. The body adjusts hormone levels to dissolve the stored fat and make it accessible by the metabolic functions or by other processes in the body. Moreover, various repair processes start to develop to re-adjust the bodily dimensions and to maintain structural regards in the body. Some changes that occur in the way of processes happening during fasting are readily more important and are as follows:

- **Human Growth Hormone (HGH)**: this is a type of hormone produced by the pituitary gland. This is significant for cellular growth and spurs growth in children and adolescents. It is very helpful in regulating body composition, body fluids, muscle and bone growth, sugar and fat digestion, and heart function also. HGH is also an active part in most of the prescription drugs in favor of growth or diseases involving weaknesses. Low production of human growth hormone could cause various diseases like Turner's syndrome which affects a girl's development, Prader-Willi syndrome, chronic kidney disease, children born small. The growth will be dismantled. But with fasting, these levels of Growth Hormones could be increased up to 5-folds. With this greater increase, this will benefit the body with muscle gain, fat loss and much more.

- **Insulin level maintaining**: Another significant hormone produced by the pancreas which allows your body to use sugar from carbohydrates eaten within the diet that is eaten for energy or to store in the body for later use. Insulin helps in keeping the sugar level from rising too high, a condition called Hyperglycemia.

Most of the cells in the body need sugar for energy. This sugar doesn't come straight from the diet. Sugar from diet comes along with insulin produced by the pancreas to enter the cells as insulin is a key to unlock the cell's membrane and energy is got by sugar inclusion. With the fasting ways, insulin sensitivity is improved and the level of insulin drop accordingly. This lower level of insulin in the blood allows accessing stored fat in the body.

- **Cellular repair**: cellular repair is a process in which different repairs tend to happen that are much needed to perform the functions of cells. Mostly, cells which are damaging and harmed due to some diet problems or chronic disorders requires a break to settle down the issues and regulate the processes. These breaks are provided by fasting methods. Whenever you fast, your cells start burning fats and start repairing their losses and regulating their functions by producing enough amount of enzymes and hormones. As a result, the processes in the body regulate to their ideal extent. Mostly, cells protect their DNA which might have been harmed before, improves alertness which impulses brain functions, skin cell repair could enhance the beauty of skin, lowers the inflammatory signs which result in stopping of disease spreads likewise the case of asthma, guaranteeing Longevity, which initiates Autophagy(cellular cleanup), improving longevity and healthy aging, hormonal improvement, and metabolic improvements.

- **Gene Expression**: genes are the encoders of protein and this encoded protein than determines the cell function. Therefore, the numbers of genes expressed in particular cells determines the functions of cells. Gene expression is the process through which information present in the gene is used to synthesize the gene product that would be purely functional. These products are mostly proteins. This process of gene expression is used by almost all organisms ranging from simple eukaryotes to complex eukaryotes. Gene expression might include several steps likewise transcription, translation, and regulation. Gene regulation provides control over cell structure and operations. It provides the basis for cell's differentiation, morphogenesis, the versatility, and adaptability of organisms. Gene regulation acts as a basis for evolutionary change by controlling the amount of gene expression, timing and location might have an impact on functions of the gene in the cells. Gene expression has a fundamental role in genetics. Therefore, regulation of gene expression has a vital role in the development of an organism. By fasting, cellular repairs might contribute to gene expression. As a consequence, improving the development of the human body.

These above-mentioned requisites are the impacts provided by fasting methods. Whenever you start fasting, within 24 hours of fasting, your body will start developing the habit of repairing and building muscles by repairing cellular operations and stimulating the growth of the cells. The stimulated growth will guarantee the growth and development in overall processes of the body and will replenish your body.

1.3. What to expect when starting to fast?

Starting to fast isn't a regular phenomenon. You need to develop some habits and build stamina to bear hunger and perform your daily tasks with fewer calories. A realistic mindset is required to start the fasting patterns or any other dietary plans. A realistic mindset is the outcome of realistic expectations. These realistic expectations might motivate you for futuristic fasting experiments. If one starts fasting without realistic and right expectations and will end up not meeting them. He/she will be discouraged and will end up quitting straight away. On the other hand, if you start with too low expectations, you will never be motivated enough to start fasting.

Your expectations might focus on different dimensions and areas, depending on what you want from your dietary plan, fasting or life-changing activity. You must be packed with some ideas to reach the target limits and adopt the right approach to reach there. Some realistic expectations might have some reasons behind and must be feasible. Some of these expectations are discussed in further paragraphs:

- Stamina building for Hunger: hunger is adopted with regular patterns in fasting. This must be kept in mind while starting to fast. The fasting process requires stamina for hunger in the long run. This stamina must be a part of expectations from fasting. Whatever you expect from fasting could devise the strategy to adopt for fasting. At the start, try using shorter periods for fasting. This will help you in developing the habit of fasting. As the habit develops, you may go on with increasing the timespan and raise your stamina to a higher proportion. As time goes on, this stamina building will help you in fasting for longer periods and benefiting the body at large from fasting

- Losing fat: losing fat is a primary goal and expectation from fasting. This requires pre-set goals to determine what amount of fat loss is feasible for you. This might be set on losing a pound a week ratio. This way, by going with the plan and meeting the expectations, the overweight person could lose 4 to 5 pounds in 30-day timespan which is a fair way to go through. Fasting, being a proven exercise, could be a greater way to lose your fats and lose weight. It could help one to get there more quickly rather than any other diet plan or method. But one must accept the fact that it takes time to lose fat and lose weight. Don't think that you start fasting and lose weight overnight. It will take a while to burn excess fat and lose weight. There are no quick ways to get through to the ideal weight.

- Feeling Healthier: a difficult thing to describe is feeling healthier. Because healthy feelings are different from person to person. When you feel healthier, you will definitely know it. You will notice being lighter on your instincts and working would be a lot safe and sound together with joys and pleasures. Talking about the joints in your body, you will feel like having springs in your joints. The dusty substance in your mind will start to leave and you will feel enthusiastic while working on your processes. Your concentration will start flourishing and you will feel better on your work and daily life routine.

- Being more energetic: being on fasting will enthusiast your feelings and will enlighten your thoughts together with enthusiasm. It will leave you more energetic, more alert by losing your weight, feeling lighter, and less irritable. You will have more energies to perform the activities you love and go out with your friends and family. Losing weight and feeling more energetic could be the thought you have developed in your strategy to go on with fasting and approach would be quite significant.

1.4. The Right Mindset and Approach

Fasting requires some out of the box approaches to tackle the demands and be realistic with the requirements. If someone is willing to opt for fasting and adopting the type of fasting, say intermittent fasting to build the physique or lessening the abdomen to lose weight, he/she must act accordingly, must prepare a plan to follow heartedly and enjoy the benefits at the end. People love to start fasting but don't think about the groundwork necessary to initiate the fasting cycle. This results in loss of health and diseases might take over the body, resulting in weakness and mental discomfort together with more expenses on health. People often see it as okay to imitate their close friends, relatives, and blood relations. They may be trying something fishy that, on imitating, may not suit their health or may not be a good condition for their body. This results in various mishaps that might cause disruption in your life.

The right mindset is actually making proper planning, implementing that plan and enthusiasting the mind to act according to that plan, sticking to the plan while moving ahead in life. Talking about the right mindset and approach to adopt while going to perform intermittent fasting, could be increasingly popular eating patterns that not only involves immediate eating cuts or restricting food intakes but also involves a proper pattern to follow while eating in 24-hour time span or in a week. This will come out with a range of health benefits, likewise increase in Human Growth Hormone (HGH) and genetic expressions. These are possible with longevity and might result in a lowered risk of diseases. Therefore, a person who performs intermittent fasting regularly will hope to live longer, healthier and lose weight.

More elaborately, insulin levels in blood drops which results in fat burning and consequently losing weight. Growth hormone level increases up to the 5-folds in blood and results in fat burning and muscle gains. It also caters more benefits. With the continuous fasting procedure, body induces major cellular repairs like excreting waste materials from cells and applaud genetic expression via beneficial changes in genes and molecules related to longevity and protection against diseases.

Setting aside these benefits, let's proceed with the topic under consideration that is the right mindset and right approach towards intermittent fasting. The right mindset, as mentioned above, is proper planning and setting goals from the fasting cycle. This involves a cycle of fasting period in between 24 hours to one week, depending upon your stamina and physique. At first, analyze your body conditions and describe the physical characters of your body, likewise, the surplus fats, the shape of your body, either belly type or skinny, etc. These all will decide about your minimalistic approach towards intermittent fasting. If you have defined your body condition, the next step is to formulate a plan or strategize your fasting according to your needs or requirements. Opt from different methods of fasting that best suits your physique and act accordingly.

Some most common and famous methods to follow include the 16/8 method which is also called the Lean gains protocol. This condition involves skipping of breakfast for fasting purposes. But do opt this technique if you have built stamina of fasting 16 hours between the meals. The person following this method skips the breakfast and restrict his/her eating period to 8 hours, convenient to his daily routine, such as 1 to 9 p.m. after this eating timespan, he/she starts fasting for 16 hours from 9 p.m. to 1 p.m. next day noon. This methods require stamina boost and also develops stamina habit in the body due to the longer period of fasting. This longer timespan and shorter eating time will make you eligible for health benefits and enthusiasts your health towards perfection.

Another method for fasting is the eat-stop-eat method which involves fasting for 24 hours timespan, once or twice in a week, depending upon your body conditions and needs of your body. This involves setting a meal as a starter of fasting. For example, eating dinner in night one day and then fasting till the next day dinner. This requires a lot of stamina and bearing power because it might result in weakness, routine disturbance, and work disturbances. Being on starvation for a whole day will leave you prone to weakness if you are not fully prepared for this. Try to adopt this approach if you are mentally and physically prepared for this. In case of a no, don't try to opt this.

The third method is the 5/2 diet method that involves consuming 500-600 calories of diet on two non-consecutive days in a week. Thus providing plenty of time to settle down your body conditions and doesn't need a special diet plan or comprehensive approach towards what to eat in this phenomenon. Therefore, it offers more flexibility and requires less attention with less involvement of your body and rewards also less than other techniques of intermittent fasting. This technique allows it, user or curator, to eat normally on other 5 days of the week. Therefore, offers more joys with fewer efforts.

The right approach is adopting the right way to

perform intermittent fasting and then moving ahead with that method and eating pattern followed according to the prescribed phenomenon. The right approach also involves what to eat and how to pass those fasting hours, either by indulging in hard works or duties or performing soft duties to prevent the body from dehydration and hunger. The more realistic you are in fasting, the more beneficial it will be for your body. With these elaborated realistic approaches, one might get maximum benefits from these fasting methods.

CHAPTER 2

Different Ways To Accomplish Intermittent Fasting And Their Pros And Cons

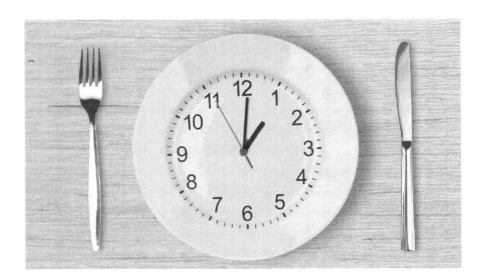

Intermittent fasting is accomplished with various methods and implemented those plans to perform intermittent fasting and acquire your desired results. These methods re extensively elaborated in the following paragraphs.

2.1. The 16:8 Method of Intermittent Fasting

This is one of the famous fasting methods, involves

limited consumption of food and limited calorie-containing foods and beverages to set eight hours' time frame per day and restricting yourself from food for remaining 16 hours in the day. Depending upon your stamina, this cycle of food ingestion and restraint can be repeated as frequently as you like. This may vary from once or twice per week to everyday and depends on your personal needs and preferences. This method has got a boost in its popularity in recent years. It popularity mostly lies among people who want to lose weight and burn fat with convenience and ease and as early as possible. Another fact for weight loss techniques, nutritionists might put extensive restrictions, strict rules, and regulations. Whereas this method is quite simple with no restrictions on what to eat and how much to eat. It is quite easy to follow and provides maximum results with minimum efforts.

Talking more about the outcomes of intermittent fasting, it is believed to improve blood sugar control, boost brain function and longevity. A problem with this method is you are not making decisions based on how much hungry you feel but on a restricted time frame. Mostly, people do this by starting fast at night, skipping breakfast, and eating the first meal in the middle of the day at about 1 p.m. No restrictions on some kinds of food are mentioned. It is left to the person who is going to adopt this method to follow a specific diet plan or adopting simpler to eat method. Now moving ahead, let's have some knowledge about how to start intermittent fasting.

2.1.1. How to get started with 16:8 method?

16/8 method of intermittent fasting is simple, safe, fantastic and sustainable. To get initiated with this method, pick a suitable eight-hour timespan that best suits your daily routine. Next step is to limit your food ingestion to that eight-hour timespan. Mostly, people prefer to eat between noon and 8 p.m. with fasting period starting from dinner to next day noon. This means they will need to fast overnight and skip breakfast due to the fasting time. They would eat a balanced lunch and dinner, with an option of few snacks or soft drinks throughout the day.

Some others opt to eat between 9 a.m. to 5 p.m. This way it allows a healthy breakfast but a bit late, around 9 a.m., and a normal lunch at noon and a light early dinner or snacks around 4 p.m. before starting to fast. But the best thing is you can pick the time of your choice. Another fact about this diet plan is to, try adopting small meals scenarios rather than a whole meal. Try to eat snacks spaced evenly throughout the day so as to stabilize the blood sugar level of the body and keep hunger under the shed.

2.1.2. Meal Plans For 16:8 Method

For the food, the 16/8 method provides freedom to choose any class of the food according to your desires or taste. But try avoiding foods like pancake-pizza-pringles wild and don't make lame excuses for these foods. During the eating period, one must stick to a clean, whole foods diet. Likewise a healthy whole foods diet includes Fruits, for example, apples, bananas, berries, oranges, etc. and Veggies like broccoli, cauliflower, cucumber, tomatoes, etc. and Whole grains like rice, wheat, barley, etc. and Healthy Fats containing oils, and Sources of Proteins like meat, poultry, fish, eggs, nuts, seeds, etc.

Drinking calorie-free beverages like water or

unsweetened tea and coffee, can control your hydration habits and can help control your appetite while keeping you hydrated. On the other hand, consuming junk food in eating period could ruin your efforts and positive effects, resulting from the 16/8 method of intermittent fasting. This might end up by doing more harm to your body than good.

One might say yes to clean proteins, healthy fats, carbohydrates, and healthy food sources. Try skipping the ultra-processed foods, but don't skip the delicious factor. With these eating patterns, one can eat eggs, vegetables, apple and butter, and chicken or veggie portions during the whole day with 4 hours break during the day. Various other methods also exist like standards but there is no restriction on opting these. One can make his own diet plan according to his taste.

2.1.3. Benefits of 16/8 intermittent fasting

16/8 intermittent fasting technique is quite easy to follow, flexible and sustainable in the long run. It is also convenient, can cut down on the amount of time and money one needed to cook and prepare food each week. Setting this aside and talking about health, 16/8 method caters with a large list of benefits associated with health niche. These include increased Weight loss, which means it, not only restrict your intakes to a few hours in the day but also help in cutting calories intake during the day. That is why it contributes to increased weight loss. Fasting boosts metabolism and contributes to increased weight loss.

Another plus point is improved blood sugar control, which is done by fasting through reduction of insulin level in blood by up to 31% and lowers the blood sugar level by 3-6%. In this way, it potentially reduces the risk of diabetes. Another plus point is enhanced longevity. This is not well enough proved but not denied by researchers that it enhances longevity. Intermittent fasting improves brain function that might result in improves mental health and as a consequence, the physical health and control are maintained by this scenario.

2.1.4. Drawbacks of 16/8 Intermittent Fasting Method

16/8 method is also associated with many health benefits but also comes with some drawbacks.

It may not be right or realistic for everyone. As it requires specific conditions and pre-requisites to follow before indulging in fasting. First of the list of drawbacks is, restricting intakes may result in some people eating more than usual during eating periods in an attempt to make up for hours that would be spent while fasting. This method may lead to weight gain, digestive problems, and the developing of unhealthy habits.

16/8 method may also cause short-term negative side effects when you start this method. These effects might include hunger, weakness, and fatigue. These may get vanished when you get used to it, but till then it might impact you badly. Another drawback is, intermittent fasting might affect men and women differently. It impacts or interferes with fertility and reproduction in women. Further studies and researches are conducted and planned to conduct to analyze the impacts on the reproductive health of men or women.

Try to opt for gradual progress and consider stopping or consulting with the doctors if you have any concerns or issues regarding negative impacts or symptoms. Restricting food intake might results in weaknesses, starving, and food consumption and weight gains.

Setting aside the benefits or drawbacks of this method, 16/8 intermittent fasting is generally termed as safe for adults. But must be consulted or discussed with the doctor before giving it a try. This is most crucial in case of any severe health conditions. On the other hand, this is a reliable key if you are suffering from diabetes, low blood pressure, or disorders of eating. This is not so good for women who are conceiving or those who are pregnant or breastfeeding their children. In case of any mishaps or wrongs, consult your doctor for further suggestions or solutions.

2.2. Eat-Stop-Eat Method of Intermittent Fasting

The time-oriented and time-restricted diet plans are used extensively for fasting purposes. But, now, another procedure will be explained in the following lines that are Eat-Stop-Eat method. Intermittent fasting totally looks reluctant and achievable, in general. The basic idea behind any of the technique of fasting is to go without eating. This actually involves hunger for a longer period of time that maybe 24 hours or may contain 16 hours. This might involves various questions likewise, what to eat and when to eat and what rules to follow while moving ahead with the fasting methods. This may also contain either to eat or drink according to your desires or not, or you are not allowed to eat according to your desires. These questions will be answered here in the following paragraphs.

The eat-stop-eat method is introduced by Brad Pilon, who came up with this plan while he was graduating from the University of Guelph. According to him, the Eat-Stop-Eat method involves fasting for 24 hours, twice a week and then eating in remaining days of the week while sticking to the plan and doesn't necessarily need to go for dieting. You can go for three meals per day or two, according to your plan. Overall ingestion or intake is controlled and maintained up to the level mentioned in the plan, it will be great and doesn't impact by the eating patterns, about when to eat. Brad has also implied this distinction. One must eat something healthy every day. Let's assume it may be eaten before 8 a.m. in the morning as breakfast and then fast from 8 a.m. one day to 8 a.m. the next day. In this way, one would end his/her fast after 8 a.m. the next day. This way leads to weight loss and fat burn with a simpler approach and easy to handle the process. Fasting one or two days in a week ensures the calorie deficit over the course of the week. If you eat 1600 calories normal days, you will probably lose 1600 or 3200 calories in that week by intermittent fasting. This equals to the amount you eat those days in case of no fasting.

2.2.1 How the Eat-Stop-Eat method works?

When one tries to cut down its eating window, it means that he/she trying to create a fasting pattern that entails the body to utilize its own stored glycogen and fats to fuel the body for proper working and functioning as a whole. The glycogens and glucose stored are used first and when it comes to an end, the body switches to fats that are accumulated in different parts of the body. This is termed as Ketogenic state and body start burning fats.

This method works in a fairly simple way, means one has to fast only two times a week, involving a full-fledge break from food for 24 hours continuously. This is elaborated with an example as you may eat normally till 7:00 p.m. on Saturday, then fast until 7:00 p.m. on Sunday and resume regular eating at that time. If one cannot make up to 24 hours, he/she can fast for 20 to 24 hours according to his/her stamina and bearing power.

After this timespan, consume 2000 calories a day for women and 2500 calories a day for men the next couple of days. It is highly recommended to not fast on consecutive days. After several non-fasting days, one can repeat the schedule and have another fast. Going with only one fast a week could make a deficiency of 10 percent in calorie consumption. On fasting days, one should take in as few calories as possible. Diet experts recommend only to take tea, coffee, plain water or diet soda. After completing fasting timespan, one can eat whatever he/she likes. But do consider a moderate rate while eating, because eating without checks could undo the benefits of fasting. There is no need to avoid any specific foods. It is recommended to eat fruits, vegetables, and spices. When it comes to proteins, it is highly recommended to consume 100 grams daily to meet the requirements of the body's energy levels. If one still getting weight between fasting patterns, one must cut down food consumption by 10 percent in non-fasting days.

In the Eat-Stop-Eat method, one must engage his/her body to weight training and resistance so as to build muscles and maintain ideal shape. There is no need to exercise on fasting days, it is best to exercise 3 to 4 times a week with 2 to 4 exercise per body parts, 2 to 5 sets per exercise, and 6 to 15 repetitions per set.

2.2.2   Benefits of the Eat-Stop-Eat method

The first and foremost benefit is restricting food intake only once or twice a week, and then eat whatever and whenever you want in the rest of the days. No foods are restricted and no specific foods are advised. Another benefit is time flexibility as one can start according to his/her will. One may start at 6 p.m. or 7 p.m. according to his availability and flexibility. This implies eating in the night so that one complete day didn't go without food. This only needs to do once or twice a week according to the lifestyle you make for your life. It accommodates workout, going for a party and attending family schedules or events.

This is surely a great plan to work because it only demands to focus on one or two days a week. One can halt the days according to his/her busy schedules. One may opt weekend days to fast as it may offer more flexibility, less work and less tiredness as compared to the working days of the week. One of the most significant benefits is reduced inflammation and cellular cleansing so as to work for your body efficiently. Eat-stop-eat is less confusing and more straightforward as compared to diet plans which imply limiting an entire food group, like fat or carbs.

2.2.3 Drawbacks of the Eat-Stop-Eat method

Not eating a single calorie intake commodity for as long as 24 hours could be hard to cope up. It may increase the likelihood of bingeing once the fast is over. Another drawback is only restricting your calories intake once or twice a week may not result in weight loss you are expecting if you overeat in no fasting days.

This way of fasting may cause headaches and crankiness in most people, and it may not be viable for people with diabetes, pregnant women or people with a history of eating disorders like bingeing. This plan of fasting allows sweetened drinks that might actually make you crave sweets and unhealthy foods as you have saved calories. This method doesn't make specific meal-plans for non-fasting days, leaving one to elaborate enormous self-control and decode on your own what to eat and when to eat. This is, in fact, the drawback where most people struggle for guidance on how to lose weight. If one wanna try the eat-stop-eat method of intermittent fasting, consult with your doctor first, and then try one day a week and see how it goes.

2.3. The 5:2 Method of Intermittent Fasting

Fasting is a way or pattern of eating that involves regularizing of eating habits so as to gain muscles, lose weight and shape your body. This involves a regular way of fasting to perform all the above-mentioned tasks.

The 5:2 method of intermittent fasting is also known as the Fast Diet, is currently the most popular and favorite type of intermittent fasting. It was introduced and familiarized by **British journalist Michael Mosley**. It's called the 5:2 diet because five days of the week are normal eating days, while the other two implies restrictions on calorie intake to about 500–600 per day. For example, a person who regularly eats about 2,000 calories per day would eat 500 calories on fasting days. There is no restriction on what to eat as there are no checks on food type or food content but rather checks on when you should eat the food or take your meal. This fasting way is more like concerning lifestyle. Mostly, people find it easier to try and stick to this diet plan rather than usual calorie-restricted diet plans.

Unlike the true fasting patterns, that involves eating nothing on a pre-defined set of time, this fasting technique has a goal to cut down calorie intakes on fasting days to 25 percent of the total or restrict it to one percent of the total regular intake on normal days. For example, the person who eats on normal, about 2,000 calories per day will now eat 500 calories on fasting days. Moreover, fasting days wouldn't need to be consecutive because it is mandatory to give your body the calories and required nutrients it needs to work on. People nowadays give space to their fasting days, for example, by adopting their fewer calorie days on Monday and Thursday or Wednesday and Saturday. This elaborates the flexibility of the diet. Instead of severely restricting the foods a person can eat, the 5:2 fasting method focus on calorie reduction for 2 days of the week. This will help some people to be more satisfied with this diet, as this will not imply that they are missing out all the time. The 5 remaining days of the 5:2 diet should still involve a healthful diet.

2.3.1   How to do the 5:2 Diet?

There is no righteous way to eat on fasting days because everyone's body might respond differently to fasting. The basic principle behind is that on fast days, a person consumes just 25 percent of his normal calorie intake. The 5:2 diet, famously called **The Fast Diet**, is the most popular intermittent fasting diet nowadays.

The 5:2 diet is basically very simple to explain. For

five days of the week, you can eat normally and don't need to think about restricting calories. Then, for the other two days of the week, you lessen up your calorie intake to a quarter of your daily requirements. This is actually about 500 calories per day for women and 600 calories per day for men. These two days wouldn't need to be consecutive. A more fundamental and easy way to plan and have restricted diet is to fast on Monday and Thursday or Wednesday and Saturday, with two small meals on the day, and then to eat normally on remaining days of the week. This is significant to emphasize on an eating pattern that eating normally doesn't mean that you can eat junk foods or binge on junk foods, this way you won't lose weight and you might get adverse effects of weight gain. You must respect your normal eating pattern as it was in no fasting days.

There is no righteous or standard way to eat on fasting days, as everyone's body may respond differently to fasting. Some people initiate the day with a small breakfast to get going or get to their bodies moving. For some others, eating breakfast might make them feel hungry throughout the day.

Those people try to wait as long as possible before their first meal of the day. Therefore, everyone's diet plan might look different. Some fast day diet plans might include:

- eating three small meals like an early breakfast, afternoon lunch, and late dinner
- eating an early lunch and dinner
- eating a small breakfast but late lunch and skipping dinner
- eating a single meal throughout the day at dinner or breakfast

2.3.2   What to eat on Fasting days?

A person can eat variety and class of foods to meet his calorie needs or requirements. These foods include a considerable part of vegetables, yogurt, eggs, fish or lean meat, cauliflower rice, soups, low-calorie soups, coffee, tea, and water. It is vital to keep the body groomed on fast days by eating foods that are rich in fiber and protein. For this purpose, eating more vegetables may help those who just started. Vegetables are very low in calories comparing to animal products and grains.

Protein is significant for staying accommodated during fast days. One must focus on taking lean sources of protein catering less fat. Add small portions of proteins on fast days in the diet. Most of the fruits are rich in natural sugar content, such as blackberries and blueberries, may contribute to sweet cravings without adding many calories. Other foods to include in this scenario are Soup which is a great food for fasting patterns, as the water and spices might help a person feel more satisfied without eating too many calories. Water is vital every day, but during fast days it might help prolong the time between meals and plain, unsweetened coffee and tea are bearable during fast days.

To restrain extra calories or accommodating the daily calorie limit on foods with fewer nutritional benefits, a person must avoid the following foods on fast days:

Processed foods, refined carbohydrates and excess fats like oils and cheese.

2.3.3   Health benefits of 5:2 Diet

There are a few studies and researches on the 5:2 diet specifically. But not in the case of intermittent fasting. There are a bunch of studies on intermittent fasting in general, which have verified impressive and enthusiastic health benefits.

- One significant and fundamental benefit is that intermittent fasting is easier to follow than continuous calorie restrictions or diet plans, at least for some people.
- Many pieces of research have confirmed that different types of intermittent fasting will considerably reduce insulin levels.
- One of those studies has shown that the 5:2 diet has actually caused weight loss similar to regular calorie restrictions or diet plans. This weight loss property is, in fact, the cause of adopting intermittent fasting and specifically 5:2 method. To lose weight, a person must eat lesser calories than he actually burns. This is known as a caloric deficit. When someone follows it accordingly and correctly, the 5:2 diet may be a simple, straightforward way to cut calories.

- This diet is in fact very effective in reducing insulin levels and improving insulin sensitivity.
- Some studies have judged the health effects of modified alternate-day fasting, which is very similar to the 5:2 diet and is commonly called 4:3 diet. It helps reduce insulin resistance, asthma, seasonal allergies, heart arrhythmias, menopausal hot flashes and more.

After 12 weeks of successful fasting, the fasting group had:

- Reduced body weight by above 11 pounds (5 kg).
- Lessened up fat mass by 7.7 pounds (3.5 kg).
- Reduced blood levels of triglycerides by 20%.
- Increased LDL particle size, which is a good thing.
- Decreased levels of leptin by up to 40%.

To opt for better choices for health and weight loss, it is basically not feasible for many of us to restrict our food intake for multiple days in a week. Life is way too short to exempt the number of days you're "allowed" to eat in a calendar year from 365 to 261, especially if it restricts you from doing other beneficial things, like having a regular exercise, going out and enjoying meals with people you love. There is even more to nourishment than calories, so do pay attention to that before buying into any trendy diet or eating plan. Be there if you are getting the benefits you desired and trendy outcomes.

CHAPTER 3

What To Get And How To Get From
Intermittent Fasting

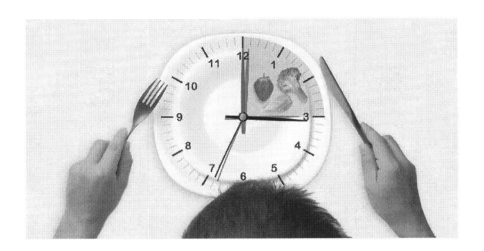

3.1   Intermittent Fasting and Weight Loss

If you are in dire need of losing fat, intermittent fasting is the perfect tool for you. Researches have shown that intermittent fasting through interchanging start and end periods of fasting and non-fasting has huge benefits for your body and brain. It can be written off chronic disease, improve memory and brain functions, and boost your energy levels. Intermittent fasting is a powerful package for losing weight quickly and keeping it for a long time.

It has the ability to fast-track your weight loss goals by eradicating accumulated fat, reducing calories, and replenishing your metabolism for better performance.

When you opt to do intermittent fasting, you eat total calories your body needs but in a shorter period of time. There are many ways to perform this fasting, but the most common of them involves eating during a 6-8 hour fasting window and going for fasting for the remaining 14 to 16 hours. It is not as hard as it looks like, especially in that case if you add Bulletproof Coffee to keep hunger levels in check.

Some research studies have shown that intermittent fasting steers weight loss at a faster pace. In a 2015 survey pool of 40 different studies, participants put light on losing on average 10 pounds in a 10-week period. Another study has found out that the adults following an "alternate day" intermittent fasting schedule or in fact eating 25 percent of their daily calories in one day, and eating normally the following day, have lost up to 13 pounds over 8 weeks period.

Intermittent fasting also gets success where many

weight-loss methods fail, by calmingly targeting and reducing accumulated fat. The accumulated fat is the internal fat layered deep around your abdominal organs. During a period of six months, people trying intermittent fasting diet became able to decrease four to seven percent of their accumulated, surplus fat.

If you are worried about its feasibility, fasting is not that unnatural. Your ancestors or humans in the past evolved to tackle miserably the situations when food deficiencies took place. On top of the stack of other health benefits, intermittent fasting steers a perfect storm of metabolic changes to tackle weight loss and fat reduction. But the question is that how does it work?

This works by tackling a variety of issues and kick-starting boosters Ketosis, lowering insulin levels, improving cholesterol, reducing inflammation and boosting metabolism.

- o Initiating Ketosis: Reaching full ketosis requires careful planning and extreme carbohydrates limiting, but intermittent fasting proves to be a shortcut to this fat dissolving state. Once your body starts draining glucose that is the actual primary source of energy then it implies to use its fat reserves for energy involving a process called ketosis. Ketosis improves the chemistry of the blood, helps in reduces inflammation, and in return helps your body in rapid weight loss.

o Helps in lowering insulin levels: Intermittent fasting implies the action of insulin in two ways. At first, it boosts your adiponectin levels, which is vital in restoring insulin sensitivity to prevent weight gain and diabetes. At second, fasting helps in decreasing fasting insulin levels. Lowered insulin is, in fact, the key your body needs to switch the mode to burning accumulated fat instead of glucose.

o Improves cholesterol: Intermittent fasting diets influence the formation of cholesterol by decreasing levels of LDL and VLDL cholesterols, both are considered bad ones.

o Helps in reducing inflammation: Lowered levels of inflammation are vital in losing weight, enhancing longevity, and eliminating the risk of major illnesses such as Alzheimer's and cancer.

o Helps in Boosting metabolism: Intermittent fasting allows to boost protein, fat, and glucose metabolism verified in animal studies. In this way, it helps your body burn more calories throughout the day, even when you are resting. Fasting boosts the levels of adrenaline and noradrenaline, hormones that help free up more stored energy in case of your body fat during a fast.

o Eating low-carbohydrates: restricting carbohydrates will regulate and reduce your appetite, and pave the way for your body to shift to the state of ketosis.

o Break your fast with right fat, high-quality meal: prepare healthy foods for the ending of the fast before the end so as to avoid bingeing and junk foods.

3.2. Health Benefits

Intermittent fasting caters many health benefits that drive most people towards it. These benefits serve the body as a whole and are comprehensive in nature. Some of them include:

- o Increase Your Fat Burning Hormone By 700%
- o Control Your Hunger Hormone and puts an End to Cravings
- o Decreases Your Stress Hormone so that you can Burn More Belly Fat
- o Boosts Your Brain Function For Better Memory and Concentration
- o Boosts Your Metabolism & Energy
- o Reducing the Risk of Diabetes
- o Increases your Testosterone level If You are a Man
- o Increases Insulin Sensitivity So that You Can Eat More and your body regulates insulin and you Stay Slim
- o Faster your Weight Loss pace
- o Decreases Inflammation So the Joints Heal and Feel Better
- o Helps in rapid Cleansing and Renewal of Your Body At Cellular Level

These benefits if elaborated in detail could be vital for driving masses towards intermittent fasting.

Different methods of intermittent fasting possess a

large list of **benefits** in regards to the health niche. These include **Weight loss**, which means it, not only restrict your intakes to a few hours in the day but also helps in cutting calories intake during the day. Fasting **boosts metabolism** and contributes to rapid weight loss.

Moreover, it improves **blood sugar control**, which is done by intermittent fasting through **reduction of insulin level** in blood up to 31% and lowers the blood sugar level by 3-6%. In this way, it potentially reduces the risk of diabetes. Another health benefit is enhanced longevity. This is not exactly proved but does not deny by researchers that it **enhances longevity**. Intermittent fasting **improves brain function** that might result in improves mental health and as a consequence, the physical health and control are improved by this scenario.

One of the most significant benefits is reduced inflammation and cellular cleansing so as to work for your body efficiently. It also regulates bodily functions. It helps reduce insulin resistance, asthma, seasonal allergies, heart arrhythmias, menopausal hot flashes and more like Cognitive functions improved, short periods will help digestive system in taking a rest, possesses the ability to increase lifespan of the individual by regularizing every function and organ, reduce risk of developing chronic diseases and avoid from major diseases, Improve blood pressure, metabolic rate, cholesterol level, and insulin sensitivity, and reduces the levels of IGF-1 in the blood.

3.3. Who should avoid it?

Fasting for a limited period or intermittent fasting is normally termed as safe for everyone, but in fact, the following populations shouldn't even think too fast without consulting a medical practitioner.

- People suffering from a medical condition like heart disease or type 2 diabetes. They are unable to suffer hunger and rely on starving as this may increase LDL cholesterol level or may disrupt insulin level in blood so as to disturb the glucose cycle in the body.
- Women who are planning to conceive
- Women who are pregnant or breastfeeding in the present days. These women require extra food, proper diet, or a balanced diet to keep up

to their needs and cater to the needs of their babies.

- o People with underweight conditions. They must not try intermittent fasting as it implies to lose weight and they are already underweight according to their height and standards on BMI. Therefore, they must avoid intermittent fasting and try to eat healthy foods to gain weight.

- o Those who are suffering from an experience of eating disorder must avoid intermittent fasting as they may have developed inflammation in their intestines or esophagus, which might result in more damage and more harm while remaining in hunger. Or eating disorder might get severe with starving.

- o People who suffer from the problems of blood sugar regulation. Blood sugar is vital for the body as it supplies the needed energy for the body to function properly. With this being an issue of vital importance, people who suffer from blood sugar regulation problems must not try to indulge in intermittent fasting as this result in starving and might disrupt your body's sugar level to a very low status that might harm severely to your body.

- People with low blood pressure must not try intermittent fasting as it triggers more reluctantly and viciously the problem to a higher extent and reach up to the dead-end level resulting in damages and destructions to the body.

- Those who are ingesting any type of prescription medications, they must try to avoid fasting as they will have to skip their medicines for fasting window. This will disrupt their process of treatment and cure and will trigger the disease as well.

- A woman possessing a history of amenorrhea

- Older adults, because they may lack the ability to bear hunger and suffer the starving situation. This might develop diseases in them if they go for fasting at that age.

- Adolescents

These persons must avoid fasting so as to maintain their physical situation and be on the safer side.

3.4. How to start fasting?

Various significant nutrition researches of present days suggest that you must eat less frequently, to force yourself to go for longer periods of time without food. This was a common phenomenon a few centuries back. Our basic, fundamental instincts drive our brain to function properly when we go hungry and physically active. The way many of us eat to eradicate hunger with snacks high in simple carbohydrates will leave the body craving for a constant sugar fix. Without proper food and sugar level, you crash and suffer from fatigue, mental clarity lacking and destroying athletic performance, among other things. But fasting has proven to be helpful for stabilizing blood sugar levels through a process called glucose regulation.

Fasting is totally different from a cleansing material or something juicy or a two-day restrictive diet. There are two categories for fasting. One is traditional and the other, intermittent. Each of these categories applies to different individuals depending on their goals and lifestyles. There are various steps to start fasting and how to imply it to your life might be different.

Step 1: Choosing the length of the fasting window

Intermittent fasting usually demands a long run routine making for the short term fasts that are viable for a specific part of every day and its physical affiliations and influences are way greater than that of traditional fasting. This is purely an effective one to normalize blood sugar, which paves the way of eradicating a bunch of symptoms like fatigue, mood swings, and metabolic health. Moreover, it has the ability to protect your brain from stroke, neurotoxins, epileptic seizures, and oxidative stresses. It is purely an effective way to rapidly lose weight, depending upon the fasting routine you choose.

If you adopt it to lose weight, try one of these, the 5:2 diet or alternate-day fasting. In later discussed fasting, you have to eat according to your routine that is to go for it five days a week, then eat up to 600 calories a day for remaining two days of the week. In upcoming days, you will continue to shift between regular and 600-calorie days. You will definitely eat fewer calories than on a normal diet, even if you keep on following your regular diet on the non-fasting days. Though it is viciously influential for those who are willing to shed a few pounds. These two styles of fasting should not be mobilized by most athletes, because you won't be eating enough calories to train properly.

Time-restricted and time-oriented fasting, also known as Leangains, is the feasible choice for persons who are looking to perform well. Eat the same amount of food you normally eat but eat it in a shorter timeframe, ideally eight hours to eat and sixteen hours for fasting. You will expect various benefits of fasting without even cutting down your calorie intake, which will make you keep training hard. It is, therefore, easy to maintain your weight or gain lean mass.

With time-bound eating, your goal is to fast for at least 12 hours a day, which is the key point from where the benefits of fasting begin. Pick the time frame that best possibly suits your life. Most of the people choose to eat from the noontime through dinnertime because it seems a lot easier to incorporate into a regular family and social life. It is viable to train yourself during the part of the day when you are not eating. Many people will try to set their training for hunger after they have eaten some food, often after work. While 12 hours for fasting seems like a reasonable timeframe to not eat food even when you aren't fasting, this implies no late dinner reservations, no snacks at the Friday night movie, and no early morning coffee when you wake up to perform morning workout. And if it really feels easy to eat only in a 12-hour window, try decreasing it up so that you would become able to go for only eight hours a day.

Step 2: Choosing the time of the fasting window

Intermittent fasting is a cycle between eating food and abstaining from food within a pre-defined window of time. The length and frequency of your fasting time schedule will depend on the approach you take. The question under discussion here is How Often Can You Fast? Here Four Intermittent Fasting Schedules are mentioned below to know much about the time and length of the fasting window.

- o Daily Time Window for Fasting

A daily schedule for fasting involves eating within a certain period of time, normally lasting 8 to 10 hours, and the whole 7 days of the week. A method like this is commonly known as 16/8 fasting, which involves eating all of the day's meals within eight hours, then abstaining from food for the remaining 16 hours of the day. For example, a person is reluctantly able to eat breakfast at 10 a.m. and eating dinner at 6 p.m., then fast until breakfast the next day.

If you are a beginner to fasting, you might consider increasing the length of your eating time window. Start with 10 hours, for example, eat breakfast at 9 a.m. in the morning and dinner at 7 p.m. in the evening and move ahead with this. The persons who are experienced with fasting might prolong the fasting window up to 20-hour fasts, eating within just a four-hour time frame. With this daily fasting schedule, consistency matters more than the length of your eating window. Experienced fasters might eat one large meal per day (23:1 hours ratio for fasting during the whole day), while an individual just initiating the fasting dilemma may eat within 10 hours. The key characteristic is to repeat the same cycle of fasting and eating periods each day of the week.

- o Daily fasting window schedules

Try out these listed schedules, selecting the eating plan that proves to be best for your lifestyle and experience with fasting. Remember to repeat the same cycle every day with the regular time frame and abiding by that time frame.

- ❖ 14:10, eat period is between 9 a.m. – 7 p.m. while the fasting is between 7 p.m. – 9 a.m. the next day.
- ❖ 16:8, eat period is between 10 a.m. – 6 p.m. while the fasting period is between 6 p.m. – 9 a.m. the next day
- ❖ 20:4, this implies the eating period between 12 p.m. – 4 p.m., fasting in between 4 p.m. – 12 p.m. the next day
- ❖ 23:1, eat one big meal per day in an hour, and at whatever hour you wish
- o Skipping Meals

If you are a beginner in intermittent fasting and the practice intimidates you, a good way out is to skip meals. If you eat a well-balanced dinner, try skipping breakfast. If you are busy during the mid of the day, skip lunch and eat an early dinner. While conventional ways out recommend never to skip meals and label the breakfast as the "most important meal of the day." Now today's researches are questioning these beliefs. Skipping the meals along the day have the ability to boost your metabolism. It looks familiar like skipping breakfast could be just as beneficial as skipping dinner. When you skip one meal, do pay extra care at not overeating at the next. The goal behind this skipping meals is to become a controlled eater eating only when you are hungry. It is not an excuse to binge at your next sit-down meal or practice other forms of disordered eating.

o   Skipping meals schedule

If you choose to skip meals rather than going for a regular fasting schedule, you're eating schedule may look different each day of the week. Start with skipping one meal when you are not hungry, then look forward to skipping several meals at different time throughout the week.

- ❖ Skip breakfast: Eat only lunch and dinner
- ❖ Skip lunch: Eat breakfast, fast for the whole day, then eat dinner
- ❖ Skip dinner: Enjoy breakfast and lunch then do an overnight fast.
  - ○ Fasting on Alternate Days

Alternate-day fasting entails the schedule of fasting one day and then eating regularly the next day. On this schedule, your calorie intake for fasting days will be around 25% of your usual calories. For example, if you normally eat a 2,000 calorie diet, you will opt to limit your calorie intake to 500 calories during your fasting time. In researches done by the National Institute of Health, there are way more success stories linked with alternate-day fasts. In fact, alternate-day fasting proves to be as more effective than calorie restriction or opting for a consistent low-calorie diet. It also proves to increase life span, maintain muscle mass and decrease inflammation.

- ○ Alternate-day fasting schedule

Sticking to an alternate-day fasting schedule, just follow the cycle outlined below. You can start any day of the week as long as the cycle remains the same. Try to keep the cycle going throughout the entire week.

- ❖ Day 1: Eat 25% of normal calories intake (roughly 500 calories throughout the day)
- ❖ Day 2: Eat 1,600 – 2,000 calories
- ❖ Day 3: Eat 25% of normal day calorie intake (roughly 500 calories throughout the day)
- ❖ Day 4: Eat 1,600 – 2,000 calories
- o 24-hours fasting time frame

For a 24-hour fast (also called Eat-Stop-Eat method), you will select only one day per week and did not eat a single calorie on that particular day every week. For example, you could have your breakfast at 7 a.m. on Mondays, then not eat until 7 a.m. on Tuesdays. If this looks unbearable to you, you could opt to eat in the middle of the day, around 2 p.m., so that it does not feel as you are going an entire day without eating. The 24-hour fasting approach is proven to be extremely effective at losing body fat. Most people only do one 24-hour fast per week. Those who get experienced with fasting may choose up to two separate days per week to conduct a 24-hour fast.

- 24-hour fasting schedule

To complete a 24-hour fast, choose the day in which you most probably are less physically active. Perhaps going for opting a rest day from the gym, or a day when you are going to do light yoga rather than hard physical exercise. A fast schedule might include:

- ❖ Sunday: Eat 1,600 – 2,000 calories and conduct regular physical activity.
- ❖ Monday: Eat lunch at noon, fast for the remaining portion of the day. Take a rest from the gym.
- ❖ Tuesday: Fast through breakfast, eat lunch and conclude your fast. Resume physical activity and eat dinner as usual.

Step 3: Working on Consistency

Now everything is clear about how to implement an intermittent fasting schedule, here, it raises a question: How often should you fast?

The answer varies from individual to individual. Most individuals implement the above schedules every week or every other week. If you are a beginner to fasting, start with a moderate schedule, try to perform it every other week or every three weeks. If your body adapts well or becomes habitual, then aim for a regular, weekly schedule. This will imply consistency in your fasting periods and time frame and your body will develop your posture and working schedules according to that fasting schedule.

Pay close attention to how your body responds to your fasting schedule, and adjust as needed. Keep in mind that life changes can happen. You may need to twist around your schedule to allow for social gatherings, vacations, and physical activity or competition. Keep it as simple as you can to develop consistency and become habitual of fasting. This could only be done by adopting consistent means in the way of fasting and letting your body develop consistent dilemma for the fasting schedules.

Step 4: Extend the window if necessary

I am very aware that the mentioning of the term fasting might terrify many people, thinking about the happenings of intense suffering and starvation. They assume themselves waking up in the morning and starting their 24-hour fasting window, anxiously counting down the milliseconds until they can have the first bite of their post-fast meal. Most of the others can't even fathom the idea of going a full day without food.

It really doesn't need to be so awkward, and there is an approach that actually makes it quite doable. In fact, it's what is adopted by most of the public. It is a bit of a cheat, but it doesn't lessen the benefits of your fast. The day before your 1-Day Fast is your 1-Day Feast. On that feast day, about 3 hours after you've enjoyed the last bite of your last meal for the day, start the timer at that time for your 1-Day Fast.

For example, if you ate a big dinner around 7 p.m., your body would indulge in a "semi-fasted" state when the time is 10 p.m. Consider that the starting of your fast. Sleep for 7 to 8 hours. When you wake up, you've completed one-third of your day fast without batting an eyelash.

If you're anything like me, you might not feel hungry in the morning. There's a good chance this will happen considering how much you stuffed yourself the day before. So much for breakfast. If you can make it to lunch on a few glasses of water, then you've just knocked out 14 hours of your fast. This way the fasting window is extended up to your bearing capacity. If you can make up to at least 4 p.m., that's 18 hours. You're really on fire at this point. As the time window is extended to about 18 hours. Maybe you take a cup of peppermint tea as a reward. After all, this is when the massive health benefits from your short-term fast really start to pore in.

At this point, if you really can't take it, you can have a smoothie or smaller meal to break your fast. However, if you really want to win, continue through to dinner without taking a bite. Once you reach 10 p.m., you did a marvelous job. You have successfully completed your fast and you can go to bed dreaming about breakfast.

If you can't wait until morning to eat, the best recommendations are a small high-protein meal or, better yet, a protein shake with a few carbohydrates about an hour before you go to sleep. That way, you supply essential proteins to your muscles, while keeping your tummy satisfied until morning. The 1-Day Fast isn't easy, but it is not a kind of impossible thing, and when you stay focused on the benefits, it becomes a lot more doable. Could you do this? I bet you can and you will be.

What makes it a whole lot easier is simply making the decision to do it and determination with courage. Most people suffer from a tough time without food because they are constantly thinking about what they will eat next. In the middle of a stressful day, that just turn someone unable to handle, as the satisfaction that comes from a delicious meal sounds good, helps people soothe their blues away. When that food isn't there, they start panicking.

When you consciously make the decision that tomorrow will be a fast day, you may push to initiate a new mechanism inside yourself. You are forced to let your innards recharge while you reflect on the bad eating habits to which you have been self-medicating. Fasting is a profound tool for deep changes to happen. No wonder why people have been turning to it for centuries.

There you go. That's all you need to start intermittent fasting.

3.5. How to Fast Safely: 10 Helpful Tips

There are many different ways to fast. Intermittent fasting is an increasingly popular eating pattern which involves not eating or sharply restricting your food intake for certain periods of time. This fasting method has been linked to a range of potential health benefits, including short-term increases in human growth hormone (HGH) and changes to gene expression. Such effects are linked to longevity and a lower risk of disease. Thus, people who fast regularly often hope to lose weight or live a healthier, longer life. However, fasting can be dangerous if not done properly. Here are the tips to help you fast safely.

o Keep Fasting Periods Short

There is no single way to fast, meaning that the duration of your fast is up to you. Popular fasting windows include:

The 5:2 Pattern: Restrict your calorie intake for two days per week (500 calories per day for women and 600 for men).

The 6:1 Pattern: This pattern is similar to the 5:2,

but there's only one day of reduced calorie intake instead of two.

"Eat Stop Eat": A 24-hour complete fast 1–2 times per week.

The 16:8 Pattern: This pattern involves only consuming food in an eight-hour window and fasting for 16 hours a day, every day of the week.

Most of these regimens advise short fast periods of 8–24 hours. However, some people choose to undertake much longer fasts of 48 and even up to 72 hours. Longer fast periods increase your risk of problems associated with fasting. This includes dehydration, irritability, mood changes, fainting, hunger, a lack of energy and being unable to focus. The best way to avoid these side effects is to stick to shorter fasting periods of up to 24 hours especially when you're just starting out. If you want to increase your fasting period to more than 72 hours, you should seek medical supervision. Longer periods of fasting increase your risk of side effects, such as dehydration, dizziness and fainting. To reduce your risk, keep your fasting periods short.

○ Eat a Small Amount on Fast Days

In general, fasting involves the removal of some or all food and drink for a period of time.

Although you can remove food altogether on fast days, some fasting patterns like the 5:2 diet allow you to consume up to around 25% of your calorie requirements in a day. If you want to try fasting, restricting your calories so that you still eat small amounts on your fast days may be a safer option than doing a full-blown fast. This approach may help reduce some of the risks associated with fasting, such as feeling faint, hungry and unfocused. It may also make fasting more sustainable since you likely won't feel as hungry. Eating a small amount on fast days rather than cutting out all food may reduce your risk of side effects and help keep hunger at bay.

○ Stay Hydrated

Mild dehydration can result in fatigue, dry mouth, thirst and headaches so, it is vital to drink enough fluid on a fast. Most health authorities recommend the 8x8 rule eight 8-ounce glasses (just under 2 liters in total) of fluid every day, to stay hydrated.

However, the actual amount of fluid you need although likely in this range is quite individual. Because you get around 20–30% of the fluid your body needs from food, it's quite easy to get dehydrated while on a fast. During a fast, many people aim to drink 8.5–13 cups (2–3 liters) of water over the course of the day. However, your thirst should tell you when you need to drink more, so listen to your body. As you meet some of your daily fluid needs through food, you can get dehydrated while fasting. To prevent this, listen to your body and drink when thirsty.

- o Go for Walks or Meditate

Avoiding eating on fast days can be difficult, especially if you are feeling bored and hungry. One way to avoid unintentionally breaking your fast is to keep busy. Activities that may distract you from hunger but don't use up too much energy include walking and meditating. However, any activity that's calming and not too strenuous would keep your mind engaged. You could take a bath, read a book or listen to a podcast. Keeping busy with low-intensity activities, such as walking or meditating, may make your fast days easier.

- Don't Break Fasts With a Feast

It can be tempting after a period of restriction to celebrate by eating a huge meal. However, breaking your fast with a feast could leave you feeling bloated and tired. Additionally, if you want to lose weight, feasting may harm your long-term goals by slowing down or halting your weight loss. Because your overall calorie quota impacts your weight, consuming excessive calories after a fast will reduce your calorie deficit. The best way to break a fast is to continue eating normally and get back into your regular eating routine. If you eat an unusually large meal after your fast day, you may end up feeling tired and bloated. Try easing gently back into your normal food routine instead.

- Stop Fasting If You Feel Unwell

During a fast, you may feel a little tired, hungry and irritable but you should never feel unwell.

To keep yourself safe, especially if you are new to fasting, consider limiting your fast periods to 24 hours or fewer and keeping a snack on hand in case you start to feel faint or ill. If you do become ill or are concerned about your health, make sure you stop fasting straight away. Some signs that you should stop your fast and seek medical help include tiredness or weakness that prevents you from carrying out daily tasks, as well as unexpected feelings of sickness and discomfort. You may feel a little tired or irritable during your fast, but if you start to feel unwell, you should stop fasting immediately.

- ○ Eat Enough Protein

Many people start fasting as a way to try to lose weight. However, being in a calorie deficit can cause you to lose muscle in addition to fat. One way to minimize your muscle loss while fasting is to ensure you are eating enough protein on the days you eat. Additionally, if you are eating small amounts on fast days, including some protein could offer other benefits, including managing your hunger. Some studies suggest that consuming around 30% of a meal's calories from protein can significantly reduce your appetite. Therefore, eating some protein on fast days could help offset some of fasting's side effects.

Having enough protein during your fast may help minimize muscle loss and keep your appetite in check.

- Eat Plenty of Whole Foods on Non-Fasting Days

Most people who fast are trying to improve their health. Even though fasting involves abstaining from food, it is still important to maintain a healthy lifestyle on days when you are not fasting. Healthy diets based on whole foods are linked to a wide range of health benefits, including a reduced risk of cancer, heart disease and other chronic. You can make sure your diet remains healthy by choosing whole foods like meat, fish, eggs, vegetables, fruits and legumes when you eat. Eating whole foods when you aren't fasting may improve your health and keep you well during a fast.

- Consider Supplements

If you fast regularly, you may miss out on essential nutrients. This is because regularly eating fewer calories makes it harder to meet your nutritional needs. In fact, people following weight loss diets are more likely to be deficient in a number of essential nutrients like iron, calcium and vitamin B12. As such, those who fast regularly should consider taking a multivitamin for peace of mind and to help prevent deficiencies. That said, it's always best to get your nutrients from whole foods. Regular fasting may increase your risk of nutritional deficiencies, especially if you are in a calorie deficit. For this reason, some people choose to take a multivitamin.

- o Keep Exercise Mild

Some people find that they are able to maintain their regular exercise regimen while fasting. However, if you are new to fasting, it is best to keep any exercise to a low intensity, especially at first, so you can see how you manage. Low-intensity exercises could include walking, mild yoga, gentle stretching and housework. Most importantly, listen to your body and rest if you struggle to exercise while fasting.

CHAPTER 4

Elaborations/Derivations of Different Ways of Intermittent Fasting

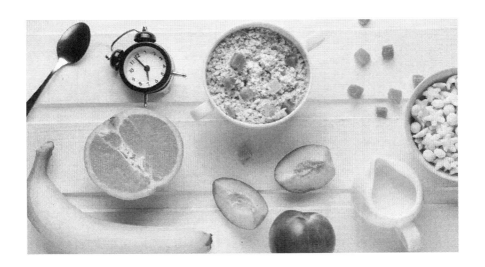

There are various ways to perform intermittent fasting, and there is no defined single plan that works for everyone. Individuals who try will experience the best results if they try to figure out the various styles to see which one suits their lifestyle and preferences. Regardless of the various types of intermittent fasting, going for fasting for prolonged periods when the body is unprepared can be problematic. These various forms of fasting or diet plans might not be suitable for everyone. If a person's body is prone to disordered eating, these approaches might contribute to their unhealthy relationship with food.

People with severe health conditions, including diabetes, should consult a doctor before attempting any form of fasting. To acquire the best results, it is essential to eat a healthful and balanced diet on non-fasting days. If needed, a person can seek professional help to personalize an intermittent fasting plan and avoid drawbacks.

Mostly, people are practicing fasting from thousands of years, talking about its safety, its safety depends more on who is doing the fasting rather than the way of fasting itself. People who have malabsorption, or suffering from low blood sugar, or possess other medical conditions should seek help or counseling from their healthcare provider. While most of the people can practice many fasting styles safely, extreme types of intermittent fasting, such as the Warrior Diet, might lead to inadequate intake of nutrients such as fiber, vitamins, and minerals. Therefore, people should approach this style of fasting with caution and care.

Now let's move to various methods of fasting and their elaborations to know them deeply and might get the whole out of it. For this purpose, all 3 methods of intermittent fasting are elaborated with their complete derivations and benefits.

4.1. 16:8 Method

One of the most famous fasting methods involves limited consumption of food and limited calorie-containing foods and beverages to set eight hours' time frame per day and restricting yourself from food for remaining 16 hours in the day. Depending upon your stamina, this cycle of food ingestion and restraint can be repeated as frequently as you like or as much you bear.

- **Advantages and Disadvantages**

16/8 method possesses a long list of **benefits** in regards to the health niche. These include **Weight loss**, which means it, not only restrict your intakes to a few hours in the day but also help in cutting calories intake during the day. That is why it contributes to increased weight loss. Fasting **boosts metabolism** and contributes to increased weight loss.

Another plus point is improved **blood sugar control**, which is done by fasting through **reduction of insulin level** in blood by up to 31% and lowers the blood sugar level by 3-6%. In this way, it potentially reduces the risk of diabetes. Another advantage is enhanced longevity. This is not exactly proved but does not deny by researchers that it **enhances longevity**. Intermittent fasting **improves brain function** that might result in improves mental health and as a consequence, the physical health and control are improved by this scenario.

Talking about the **Disadvantages** of 16:8 method, it is **not right or realistic** for everyone. As it requires specific conditions and pre-requisites to follow before indulging in fasting. First of the list of drawbacks is, restricting intakes may result in some people **eating more than usual** during eating periods in an attempt to make up for hours that would be spent while fasting. This method **may lead to weight gain**, **digestive problems**, and the developing of unhealthy habits.

16/8 method may also cause short-term negative

side effects when you start this method. These effects might include **hunger**, **weakness**, and **fatigue**. These may get vanished when you get used to it, but till then it might impact you badly. Another drawback is, intermittent fasting might affect men and women differently. It impacts or **interferes with fertility** and reproduction in women. Further studies and researches are conducted and planned to conduct to analyze the impacts on the reproductive health of men or women.

Try to opt for gradual progress and consider stopping or consulting with the doctors if you have any concerns or issues regarding negative impacts or symptoms. Restricting food intake might results in weaknesses, **starving**, and **food consumption** and weight gains. This is not so good for women who are conceiving or those who are pregnant or breastfeeding their children. In case of any mishaps or wrongs, consult your doctor for further suggestions or solutions.

- **What to Eat and What Not to Eat**

Talking about **what to eat**, the 16/8 method equips you with the freedom to choose any class of the food according to your desires or taste. But try to avoid junk foods like pancake-pizza-pringles wild. During the eating period, one must stick to a clean, whole foods diet. Likewise, a healthy whole foods diet includes:

- o Fruits, for example, apples, bananas, berries, oranges, etc.
- o Veggies like broccoli, cauliflower, cucumber, tomatoes, etc.
- o Whole grains like rice, wheat, barley, etc.
- o Healthy Fats containing oils, and Sources of Proteins like meat, poultry, fish, eggs, nuts, seeds, etc.
- o Drinking calorie-free beverages like water or unsweetened tea and coffee can control your hydration habits
- o clean proteins, healthy fats, carbohydrates, and healthy food sources

Let's talk about **what not to eat**, this involves foods that are prohibited because of their adverse effects on the human body both internally and externally.

- o Junk food consumed during the eating period could ruin your efforts and positive effects, resulting from the 16/8 method of intermittent fasting. This might end up by doing more harm to your body than good.

- o Try skipping the ultra-processed foods, but don't skip the delicious factor.
- o Avoiding overeating and unhealthy, unhygienic foods

These foods are must avoid to restrain your benefits and didn't overdo to not waste what you got from the fasting.

- **Recommended Foods**

Recommended foods include a large list of items that are mandatory to eat and could benefit your body with the desired result what you are expecting from the fasting patterns.

- o Water, as it is important to stay hydrated for many reasons, like for health of every major organ of the body
- o Avocado, as it is highest calorie fruit and adding a half of it to your lunch may keep you full for hours.

- Fish, Diet suggestions suggests eating at least eight ounces of fish per week.
- Cruciferous veggies, like Broccoli, Brussels sprout and cauliflower, which are full of fiber.
- Potatoes, as these are one of the most satiating foods around
- Beans and legumes, specifically low-calorie carbs, chickpeas, black beans, peas, and lentils are recommended for a healthy diet.
- Probiotics, add probiotic-rich foods like Kefir, Kombucha, or Kraut to your diet.
- Berries, sweet berries are a great source of immune-boosting vitamin C and must be a part of a healthy diet
- Eggs, a large egg has six grams of proteins and must be a part of a healthy diet.
- Nuts, may be higher in calories but contains good fat and is amazing to be a part of a healthy diet
- Whole grains, rich in fiber and protein so eating a little could go a long way in keeping you full and can rev up your metabolism.

These are the precise set of recommended foods to be a part of intermittent fasting and can provide you with a full-fledge diet needed to meets the body's requirements.

- **What to do on Fasting days**

Intermittent fasting is an eagerly popular eating pattern which involves not eating or restricting your food intake for pre-defined periods of time. This must be done with precautions and safety. Here are some tips mentioned below to fast safely.

- o Keep Fasting Periods Short: Longer fasting periods enhances the risks of problems associated with fasting. This involves dehydration, irritability, mood changes, fainting, hunger, lack of energy and being unable to focus. The best way to avoid those side effects is to stick to the shorter fasting periods of up to 24 hours if you're just starting out.
- o Eat a Small Amount on Fast Days: In general, fasting dictates the removal of some or all food and drink for a period of time. If you wanna try fasting, restrict your calories so that you still eat a little amount on your fast days may be a safer option than doing a fast without eating.

- Stay Hydrated: Dehydration might result in fatigue, dry mouth, thirst and headaches that's why one must drink much fluid on a fast. During a fast, most people think of drinking 8.5–13 cups (2–3 liters) of water during the day. However, your thirst should tell you when you need to drink more, so listen to your body.
- Go for Walks or Meditate: To avoid eating on fast days could be difficult, especially when you get bored and hungry. This could be avoided by keeping yourself busy. Some activities that might distract the mind from hunger but don't require too much energy includes walking and meditating. Some more activities that could calm and not too strenuous, would keep your mind engaged that involves taking a bath, reading a book or listening to a podcast.
- Don't Break Fasts With a Feast: Eating a large meal after the whole fast day could result in feeling tired and bloated. Try to get back to your normal food routine at a slow pace. If you have a desire to lose weight, feasting may be harmful to your long-term goals by slowing down your weight loss scenario.

- Stop Fasting If You Feel Unwell: Being in a fast, you might feel a bit tired, hungry and irritable but must not feel unwell. To keep yourself safe and sound, if you are a newbie in fasting, focus on limiting your fasting timeframe to 24 hours or less and keep a snack or something else in case you may feel faint or ill. If you feel ill or are worried about your health, stop it immediately.
- Eat Enough Protein: Mostly people start fasting to give it a try to lose weight. However, being in a calorie deficiency situation might cause to lose muscle together with fat. There is one way to minimize your muscle loss while fasting is to ensure eating enough protein on non-fasting days. If you eat small amounts on fast days, including some protein could help in managing your hunger.
- Keep Exercise Mild: Some people figure it out that they are able to maintain their regular exercise in fasting timeframe. But if you're new to fasting, then the best thing is to keep exercises to low intensity. Low-intensity exercises include walking, mild yoga, gentle

stretching, and housework. Try to listen to your body and rest if you find yourself unable to exercise while fasting.

4.2. Eat-Stop-Eat method

The eat-stop-eat method involves fasting for 24 hours, twice a week and then eating in remaining days of the week while sticking to the plan and doesn't necessarily need to go for dieting. You can go for three meals per day or two, according to your plan. Overall ingestion or intake is controlled and maintained up to the level mentioned in the plan, it will be great and doesn't impact by the eating patterns, about when to eat. Fasting one or two days in a week ensures the calorie deficit over the course of the week. If you eat 1600 calories normal days, you will probably lose 1600 or 3200 calories in that week by intermittent fasting. This equals to the amount you eat those days in case of no fasting.

- **The eat-stop-eat method is not for everyone**

Fasting for a limited period is normally termed as safe for everyone, but in fact, the following populations shouldn't even think too fast without consulting a medical practitioner.

- o People suffering from a medical condition like heart disease or type 2 diabetes
- o Women who are planning to conceive
- o Women who are pregnant or breastfeeding the present days
- o People with underweight conditions
- o Those who are suffering from the experience of an eating disorder
- o People who suffer from the problems of blood sugar regulation
- o People with low blood pressure
- o Those who are ingesting any type of prescription medications
- o A woman possessing a history of amenorrhea
- o Older adults
- o Adolescents

These persons must avoid fasting so as to maintain their situation and be on the safer side.

- **Advantages and Disadvantages**

The **advantages** include:

- o Restricting food intake only once or twice a week, and then eat whatever and whenever you want in the rest of the days.
- o No foods are restricted and no specific foods are advised.
- o Another benefit is time flexibility as one can start according to his/her will. One may start at 6 p.m. or 7 p.m. according to his/her availability and flexibility. This implies eating in the night so that one complete day didn't go without food. This only needs to do once or twice a week according to the lifestyle you make for your life.
- o It accommodates workout, going for a party and attending family schedules or events.
- o One can halt the days according to his/her busy schedules. One may opt weekend days to fast as it may offer more flexibility, less work and less tiredness as compared to the working days of the week.
- o One of the most significant benefits is reduced inflammation and cellular cleansing so as to work for your body efficiently.

- Eat-stop-eat is less confusing and more straightforward as compared to diet plans which imply limiting an entire food group, like fat or carbs.

The **disadvantages** include:

- Not eating a single calorie for as long as 24 hours could be hard to cope up.
- It may increase the likelihood of bingeing once the fast is over.
- Only restricting your calories intake once or twice a week may not result in weight loss you are expecting if you overeat in no fasting days.
- This way of fasting may cause headaches and crankiness in most people
- May not be viable for people with diabetes, pregnant women or people with a history of eating disorders like bingeing.
- This fasting technique allows sweetened drinks that might actually make you crave sweets and unhealthy foods as you have saved calories.
- It doesn't make specific meal-plans for non-fasting days

- Most people struggle for guidance on how to lose weight.

These drawbacks let's one to care about while going for the Eat-Stop-Eat method of intermittent fasting.

- **What to eat and what not to eat during the fasting phase**

During the fasting phase, it is highly recommended to rely on:

- Soft drinks, beverages
- zero calorie diets
- Plain water
- Tea or Coffee
- Low-calorie diets
- Little veggies if in a dire need to eat something

What not to eat during the fasting phase has a large list as it involves:

- Heavy meals including Proteins, carbohydrates, fats including oils
- Vitamin-rich foods
- Calorie rich foods that are tasty and caching

- Fast foods like pizza, burgers or others like this.
- Sweetened foods or foods containing sugar as a part or whole
- Artificially sweetened foods
- Try avoiding junk foods that may contribute to weight gain rather than weight loss

These food cycle must be kept in mind while going for fasting. As fasting requires a little effort and rewards more benefits if considered with wise mind and rational thoughts. Try to adopt the method that suits you rather than just picking one and starting it. One must consult doctors or nutritional experts for better recommendations on how to start and which method to start with which foods to eat and which not to eat.

- **What to eat and what not to eat after the fasting phase**

Discussing **what to eat**, the eat-stop-eat method just like other intermittent fasting methods applauds you with the freedom to choose any type or category of the food according to your desires or taste. During the eating period or non-fasting phase, one must stick to a clean, whole foods diet. A healthy, comprehensive food diet includes:

- Fruits, for example, apples, bananas, berries, oranges, etc.
- Veggies like broccoli, cauliflower, cucumber, tomatoes, etc.
- Whole grains like rice, wheat, barley, etc.
- Healthy Fats containing oils
- Sources of Proteins like meat, poultry, fish, eggs, nuts, seeds, etc.
- Drinking calorie-free beverages like water or unsweetened tea and coffee can control your hydration habits
- clean proteins, healthy fats, carbohydrates, and healthy food sources

Moving to **what not to eat** includes foods that are prohibited because of their adverse effects on the human body both internally and externally.

- Junk food consumed during the eating period could ruin your efforts and positive effects, resulting from the eat-stop-eat method of intermittent fasting. This might end up by doing more harm to your body than good.

- Try skipping the ultra-processed foods, but don't skip the delicious factor.
- Avoiding overeating and unhealthy, unhygienic foods

These foods are must avoid to restrain your benefits and didn't overdo to not waste what you have got from the fasting. These foods will leave your body to develop fats and excessive fats will get accumulated and resulting in weight gain rather than the weight loss what you are up to.

- **Recommended foods for Eat-Stop-Eat method**

Recommended foods for this method are alike to the other intermittent fasting methods, recommendations as all are based on the same idea and results in the same benefits. It includes a large list of items that are necessary to eat and could benefit your body with the desired result what you expect from the fasting patterns.

- Water, to stay hydrated is very much important for many reasons, like for health of every major organ of the body, shining skin, body requirements, tangible muscles, and blood proper formation. There is a need for 7-8 liters of water a day.

- o Fish, nutritional experts suggest eating at least eight ounces of fish per week.
- o Cruciferous veggies, like Broccoli, Brussels sprout and cauliflower, which are full of fiber and iron.
- o Potatoes, as these are one of the most satiating foods around.
- o Beans and legumes, specifically low-calorie carbs, chickpeas, black beans, peas, and lentils are recommended for a healthy diet.
- o Probiotics, add probiotic-rich foods like Kefir, Kombucha, or Kraut to your diet.
- o Berries, as sweet berries are a great source of immune-boosting vitamin C and must be a part of a healthy diet.
- o Eggs, a large egg has six grams of proteins and must be a part of a healthy diet.
- o Nuts, may be higher in calories but contains good fat and is amazing to be a part of a healthy diet

- Whole grains, rich in fiber and protein so eating a little could go a long way in keeping you full and can revolutionize your metabolism.

These are the amazing set of recommended foods to be a part of intermittent fasting and can provide you with a full-fledge diet needed to meets the body's requirements. If the body's requirements are not fulfilled in the fasting phase, it might get adverse effects to your body. Therefore, one must supply calories according to the requirements of the body. If it feels tiredness or idleness all the time, then immediately stop fasting and consult your doctor.

4.3. The 5:2 method

The 5:2 method of intermittent fasting is also known as the Fast Diet, is currently the most popular and favorite type of intermittent fasting. It's called the 5:2 diet because five days of the week are normal eating days, while the other two puts restrictions on calorie intake to about 500–600 per day. For example, a person who regularly eats about 2,000 calories per day would eat 500 calories on fasting days. There is no restriction on what to eat as there are no checks on food type or food content but rather checks on when you should eat the food or take your meal. Mostly, people find it easier to try and stick to this diet plan rather than usual calorie-restricted diet plans.

- **How does it work?**

Every single person's body might respond differently to fasting. The basic principle behind the idea of 5:2 diet is that on fast days, a person consumes just 25 percent of his normal calorie intake. The 5:2 diet, famously called **The Fast Diet**, is the most popular intermittent fasting diet nowadays.

The 5:2 diet is actually very simple to explain. For five working days of the week, you can eat normally and there is no need to think about restricting calories. While for the other two days of the week, reduce your calorie intake to a quarter of your daily requirements. This is actually about 500 calories per day for women and 600 calories per day for men. These two days wouldn't need to be consecutive. A more fundamental and easy way to plan and have restricted diet is to fast on alternate days like Monday and Thursday or Wednesday and Saturday, with two small meals on the day, and then to eat normally on remaining days of the week. Some people initiate the day with a small breakfast to get going or get to their bodies moving. For some others, eating breakfast might make them feel hungry throughout the day. People like this try to wait as long as possible before their first meal of the day. Therefore, everyone's diet plan might look different. Some fast day diet plans might include:

- eating three small meals like an early breakfast, afternoon lunch, and late dinner
- eating an early lunch and early dinner
- eating a small breakfast but late lunch and skipping dinner
- eating a single meal throughout the day at dinner or breakfast

These diet plans vary from person to person but work well according to the expectations and hopes. Let's move towards the benefits and drawbacks of this method of intermittent fasting.

- **Advantages and Disadvantages**

  There are a few studies and researches on the

5:2 diet specifically. But not in the case of intermittent fasting. There are a bunch of studies on intermittent fasting in general, which have verified impressive and enthusiastic health benefits. These health benefits include:

- Easy to follow when compared with continuous calorie restrictions or diet plans.
- Many pieces of research have confirmed that different types of intermittent fasting will considerably reduce insulin levels.
- 5:2 diet actually caused weight loss similar to regular calorie restrictions or diet plans. This weight loss property is, in fact, the cause of adopting intermittent fasting and specifically 5:2 method. To lose weight, a person must eat lesser calories than he actually burns. This is known as a caloric deficit. When someone follows it accordingly and correctly, the 5:2 diet may be a simple, straightforward way to cut calories.
- This diet is in fact very effective in reducing insulin levels and improving insulin sensitivity.
- Some studies have judged the health effects of modified alternate-day fasting, which is very

similar to the 5:2 diet and is commonly called 4:3 diet. It helps reduce insulin resistance, asthma, seasonal allergies, heart arrhythmias, menopausal hot flashes and more.

- Cognitive functions improved
- Short periods will help the digestive system in taking a rest
- Have the ability to increase the lifespan
- Reduce the risk of developing chronic diseases
- Improve blood pressure, metabolic rate, cholesterol level, and insulin sensitivity
- Reduce the levels of IGF-1 in the blood

These are the benefits that trigger the people in attracting this fasting technique and might steer more towards this one. Talking about the disadvantages it carries, these includes:

- Overeating after fasting window
- Difficulty in sleeping, bad breaths, dehydration and anxiety.
- Nutrient deficiencies due to food restrictions
- Unsustainable solution
- Less energy which might effect in less functioning in the daily routine of life

- Not suitable for type-1 disease patient, pregnant woman, children or people recovering from surgery
- Stopping from hard exercises or workouts.

These disadvantages contribute to less adoption of this method. But the benefits are more than enough to adopt this method.

- **Foods to consider and foods to avoid**

A person opting to fast can eat various categories of foods to meet his calorie needs or requirements. These foods include a considerable part of vegetables, yogurt, eggs, fish or lean meat, cauliflower rice, soups, low-calorie soups, coffee, tea and water and other foods that are rich in fiber and protein. Vegetables are very low in calories comparing to animal products and grains.

Protein is significant for staying accommodated during fast days. One must focus on taking lean sources of protein catering less fat. Add small portions of proteins on fast days in the diet. Most of the fruits are rich in natural sugar content, such as blackberries and blueberries, may contribute to sweet cravings without adding many calories. Other foods to include in this scenario are Soup which is a great food for fasting patterns, as the water and spices might help a person feel more satisfied without eating too many calories. Water, unsweetened coffee and tea are bearable during fast days.

To restrain extra calories or accommodating the daily calorie limit on foods with fewer nutritional benefits, a person **must avoid the following foods** on fast days:

Ultra-Processed foods, refined carbohydrates and excess fats like oils and cheese, junk foods, fast foods, and oil-rich foods.

- **What to do if you feel hungry**

If you feel hungry during the fast, go with these strategical points and fast according to these keys, it will wither away your hunger and keep you aligned with the fasting methods and fasting window.

- ○ Start with 12 hours: "It's very individual how well you'll feel if you just jump straight into a 16-hour fast," says Slayton. Instead, she suggests starting with 12 hours for the fasting window.

- Eat the way you normally would at first: Instead of totally interchanging your diet to eat healthier, eating more greens, fewer carbs and sugar, start by getting the right time and then change your diet.
- Make sure your breakfast is full of protein: A breakfast rich in protein has been the guarantee for less hunger throughout the day.
- Drink a lot of water when you wake up: "Oftentimes, what we think is hunger is actually thirst," explains Slayton. Because our bodies can't detect the difference. We wake up dehydrated after sleeping, it's mandatory to drink at least 16 ounces of water in the morning.
- Eat higher fat, carbohydrates rich meals at night: It will increase your blood sugar levels which will take some time to fall. Having carbohydrates in your food increases the production of serotonin in your body, that's why you will feel great.

- Switch up your timings through trial and error: The recommendations for people are to start the fast at 7 pm or 8 pm and break it at 11 am or 12 pm for the appropriate time to have a balanced and thoughtful dinner
- Don't keep changing your fasting window: Once your body has become habitual to eating at a defined time, it is hard to change. Therefore, try to stick to the time you got.
- Make sure your mornings are busy: If you are just initiating and are habitual to having breakfast right when you wake up, the best way out is to make sure your mornings are very busy.
- Focus on something you enjoy after you eat: To stop thinking about food and diverting your mind to somewhere else, it is recommended to opt for a good distraction, like a good book, movie, or cleaning up the house.
- Exercise at night: The earlier you wake up, the more hours it will be there without food. So, instead of waking up early to work out, it is recommended to post-dinner workouts.

These options if adopted with necessary precautions

could end up extending your bearing capacity and you will not fall short of fasting window.

CHAPTER 5

Intermittent Fasting and Physical Feasibilities/Requisitions

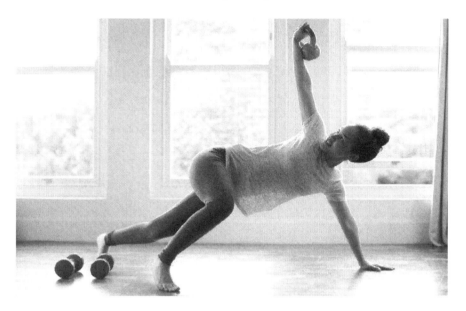

5.1.   Intermittent fasting and Workout

If you are going to try Intermittent Fasting and you still looking to get your workouts in, there are some pros and cons to consider before you decide to work out in a fasted state. Some research has proven that exercising while fasting affects muscle's biochemistry and metabolism that is joined with insulin sensitivity and the precarious control of blood sugar levels. Research supports eating and immediately exercising before digestion or absorption occurs. This is viciously important for anyone with type 2 diabetes or metabolic syndrome.

Chelsea Amengual, manager of Fitness Programming & Nutrition at Virtual Health Partners, says that advantage while fasting is that your stored carbohydrates known as glycogen, are going to be depleted, so you will be burning more fat to fuel your workout. Though, researches on this are small and countered by studies suggesting that you don't burn fat off your body when you work out on an empty stomach.

Does the news burn more fat sound like a win? While exercising in a fasted state, it is possible that your body will start breaking down muscle to use protein for fuel, plus, you are more susceptible to harms, which means you will have less energy and not be able to work out as hard or perform as well. Priya Khorana, a nutrition educator at Columbia University, believes that intermittent fasting and exercising long-term isn't ideal. Your body depletes itself of calories and energy, which could ultimately end up slowing your metabolism.

If you are ready to try Intermittent Fasting while continuing your exercise routine, there are some must-do things you can do to make your workout effective.

o   Think through timing

Registered dietician Christopher Shuff says there are three considerations when making your workout more effective while fasting: whether you should exercise before, during, or after the fueling window. Lean Gains/16:8 method is a popular method of Intermittent Fasting. This method implies to consume all food within an 8-hour eating window and then fasting for 16 hours. Working out before the window is ideal for someone who performs well going for exercise on an empty stomach, while during the fasting window is better and suitable for someone who doesn't like to exercise on an empty stomach and also conscious about capitalizing on post-workout nutrition. For performance and recovery, it is highly recommended to work out during the fasting window is the best option. After the fasting window option is for people who like to exercise after fueling/filling their stomach but don't have the opportunity to do it during the eating window.

- ○ Choose the type of workout based on your macros

It is important to pay attention to or consider the type of macronutrients you take in the day before you exercise and when you eat after exercise and fasting window. For example, strength workouts like shaping the body or muscle building, generally require more carbohydrates the day of, while cardio/HIIT [high-intensity interval training] can be done on a lower carbohydrate day.

- ○ Eat the right meals after your workout to build or maintain muscle

Dr. Son pal says the best solution for combining Intermittent Fasting and exercise is to schedule your workouts during your eating periods so your nutrition levels lie at peak. And if you do the heavy lifting, it is important for your body to eat and dissolve protein after the workout to aid with regeneration. Amengual suggests for any strength training with carbohydrates and about 20 grams of protein within 30 minutes after your workout.

- How can you safely exercise while fasting?

The success of any weight loss or exercise program depends on how safe it is to sustain over time. If your ultimate goal is to decrease body fat and maintain your fitness level while doing Intermittent Fasting, you need to stay in the safe zone. Here are some expert tips to cater you with the needs of doing that.

- ❖ Eat a meal close to your moderate- to high-intensity workout

This is where meal timing comes into play. Khorana says that timing a meal close to a moderate or high-intensity workout is key. This way your body has some glycogen stores to tap into to fuel your workout.

- ❖ Stay hydrated

Dr. Son pal says to remember fasting doesn't mean to remove water. In fact, he recommends that you drink more water while fasting to stay hydrated and fuel your body with the proper level of water so as to tackle the deficiency due to sweat.

❖ Keep your electrolytes up

A good low-calorie hydration source, says Dr. Son pal, is coconut water. It replenishes electrolytes, is low in calories, and tastes pretty good, he says. Gatorade and sports drinks rely high in sugar upon on, so avoid drinking too much of them.

❖ Keep the intensity and duration fairly low

If you indulge yourself too hard in workout and fasting and begin to feel dizzy or light-headed, take a break. Listening to your body is important. Because if your body doesn't feel well, how could you do that exercise and fasting? So, the first thing is to listen to your body and then proceed to these steps.

❖ Consider the type of fast

If you are doing a 24-hour intermittent fast, then you must stick to low-intensity workouts such as walking, restorative yoga, or gentle Pilates. But if you are continuing with the 16:8 fast, much of the 16-hour fasting window is evening, sleep, and early in the day, so sticking to a certain type of exercise isn't as critical.

❖ Listen to your body

The most important advice to pay attention or consideration when exercising during Intermittent Fasting is to listen to your body. If you start to feel weak or dizzy, chances are you're experiencing low blood sugar or prone to dehydration, explains Amengual. If that is the case, she says to opt for a carbohydrate-electrolyte drink immediately and then continue with a well-balanced meal.

While exercising and intermittent fasting may work for some people, others may not feel comfortable doing any form of exercise while fasting. Consult with your doctor or healthcare provider before starting any nutrition or exercise program.

At the end of the point, it is important to understand that what works for someone else may or may not work for you. If your workouts are only getting weaker as a result of fasting, then try twisting around with what you are eating for dinner or give a different fasting method a try or give it up altogether! Intermittent fasting might not be the right fit for your exercise or dieting goals, and that's so OK.

5.2. What is the best time to train and what are the best exercises to do?

Talking about the best exercises to do while you are with intermittent fasting contains a long list. Some of them are mentioned below briefly and shortly.

Yoga: most practitioners and trainers actually prefer to practice yoga on an empty stomach. It provides a "clean" and "light" feeling that allows you to focus entirely on your breath and body's movement. Many studios will offer early morning classes, but you can also check out Free Resource Libraries full of workouts!

Dance: dance in any form (if you enjoy it) is a fun activity that will make you completely forget about any kind of hunger. This can be in the form of ballet, barre, Zumba, hip-hop or anything else.

Tennis: if you are an avid tennis player, a morning match will be a breeze when fasted. Walking (or light jogging) put your favorite podcast on and go for a leisurely (or not so leisurely) walk or jog, anywhere from 1-4 miles.

On the treadmill: try walking on an incline (3.5 mph at an 8 incline or higher). It is actually been proven to burn more fat than jogging on a flat surface!

Cycling: whether indoors or outdoors, great music coupled with a great ride will make you feel like you are literally gliding through the air.

Pilates: similar to yoga, practitioners often prefer an empty, "light" state of being

Workouts that are to be avoided in a fasted state and must not be done in any form:

- o Boxing
- o CrossFit
- o Powerlifting
- o HIIT – classes such as Orange Theory, Barry's, etc.

Exercise routines that must be adopted while intermittent fasting and these are safe to try ad adopt:

If you've got 30 minutes:

Take a 15-minute walk (1 mile) outside or 1-mile walk on an incline on a treadmill

Spend 15 minutes with bodyweight exercises: core work, pushups, squats, and lunges

If you've got 45 minutes:

Take a 20-30 minute walk or jog (2 miles) outside or 2-mile walk on an incline on a treadmill

Spend 15 minutes flowing through a yoga workout or 15 minutes with bodyweight exercises

If you've got 1 hour:

Check what classes are available in your area, go for a bike ride or a long walk in the park. Recruit a friend to walk or bike with you, or go for a swim in the ocean or pool.

One of my favorite ways to do fasted cardio is actually spending an hour on the treadmill walking on an incline (4 miles) while catching up on my favorite shows or movies – it's actually the only time I allow myself to watch TV! Doing this genuinely makes me look forward to my 1-hour of fasted cardio.

Remember all you have to do is to be moving; what you are doing doesn't really matter, as long as it feels good to you. Make sure you stay hydrated and stop immediately if you feel weak or dizzy.

Now moving ahead with best times to train and do exercise while going together with intermittent fasting. If you are able to work out with intermittent fasting then you must schedule your work out aligned with your intermittent fasting schedule.

STEP 1: WHAT IS YOUR FASTING RATIO?

The most common fasting window is 16:8 which means you fast for 16 hours and have an 8-hour eating window. Your fasting window can be anywhere between 12-18 hours, the more hours you fast the more beneficial the fast will be for you. I like to go with the common 16:8 ratio, this way, when I work out, I am sure my body is in a fasted state.

STEP 2: WHAT TIME DO YOU WORKOUT?

Next, take into consideration the time you usually

workout at. Make sure your workout is at least an hour before you plan on breaking your fast to ensure you get the full benefits of your workout. Like I mentioned earlier, the longer you wait, the more benefits you will get. I typically try to wait 2 hours after my work out before breaking my fast.

STEP 3: HOW ABOUT THE REST OF THE DAY?

Now depending on your ratio, plan out the rest of your day and figure out what time your final meal will be at. For example, if you chose the 16:8 ratio and had your first meal at 10 am, plan to have your last meal at 6 pm.

This 3 step process will work no matter what time you choose to work out in the morning or what time you choose to break your fast, all you have to do is adjust your hours according to your schedule!

   o   Plan your meals around your workouts

Vincent recommends cardio on an empty stomach, so booking that early morning spin class or going for a jog works well if you're fasting. But choosing the right foods the night before is crucial.

Keeping in mind you are going to exercise, you should be thinking about what to eat the day before, depending on the intensity of the workout. For example, you may want to build your glycogen stores with complex carbohydrates for dinner the night before so that you have the readily available energy for a cardio workout. You never want to do cardio on a full stomach, as the sudden demand for blood flow from the muscles will steal vital blood flow needed by the digestive system for digestion and assimilation of nutrients. The key is to plan ahead so your nutrition can meet the demands required by the intensity of your workout, even when it's the next morning.

- o Which workouts should you choose?

Unless you find yourself getting lightheaded during a fast, exercise to your heart's content cardio, weight lifting, and the works. Several elite-level strength athletes state that their strength peaks after 16 or 20 hours fast. Cognitively, people tend to feel more lucid and focused while going for a workout with intermittent fasting. The more frequently you fast the easier it gets and the more benefits you'll derive from it.

If you ate a carbohydrate-centered diet for fuel, then you have to be careful about intense exercise like CrossFit, especially toward the end of a fasting period, because you may run out of fuel and feel pretty horrible like dizzy, lightheaded, nauseous, and weak. This happens when glycogen stores are depleted, which is more likely to happen when you have fasted for longer. The good news is, with less intense exercise during an intermittent fast, the body will turn to burn fat for fuel. This is great for anyone looking to trim a few inches around the waist.

As we noted above, when it comes to fasting and exercise, there is nothing more important than listening to your body. Blood sugar will drop rapidly, you may feel faint, could possibly pass out.

Sounds a little scary, right? Vincent goes into more detail, saying a little planning goes a long way.

"The most important thing to consider for people who do intermittent fasting, whether it is 14 hours or 16 hours from dinner until the first meal the next day, is what the first meal of the day is and how that fits into your exercise schedule," he says, adding that It is important to eat protein, complex carbohydrates, healthy fats, and plant-rich fibers during the eating window to maintain a healthy fast. "More complex carbohydrates are needed for workout days. More protein, plant fibers, and fats are needed on rest days."

So, there you got it. Go easy or hard, plan your meals accordingly, and most importantly, listen to your body.

If you practice intermittent fasting and do not work out in the morning, just fit your workout in wherever you can within your day. As long as you are sticking to a specific intermittent fasting schedule, you will still get a ton of benefits that come along with intermittent fasting.

5.3. How to track progress while fasting

Sometimes technology can really be our best friend and help us stick to our commitments. If you need extra support or simply want to make your life easier, there are a number of intermittent fasting apps available on the market to help you out.

Here are mentioned a number of apps and made our list of the top 6 intermittent fasting apps:

- o Zero fasting app logo Zero – The popular option for iOS users

With simple functions and simple yet elegant design, this app was one of the first on the app store and remains very popular. Set up your fasting protocol and you're good to go. Great for intermittent fasting (IF) as it gives you a notification when you've reached your goal for the day. Can also be used to track extended fasts even though the goal is limited to 24 hours.

- o Vora – The best option for Android users

Vora has always been the best option for Android users but is now also available for iOS devices. It includes several more features compared to Zeroes such as statistics of your fasts and an optional social element to it. You can log your weight and keep a fasting journal as you're going along. A great fasting tracker with everything you need.

- o Fast Habit – Another option for iOS users

Fast Habit is another iOS-only app with great design and similar features to Vora. Perhaps you've tried Zero but want more features? This is your choice.

- Body Fast
- My Fast
- Track Your Fast (Android only)

Bonus: Don't want to use an app?

If you don't want to use an app or perhaps don't own a smartphone, I'd suggest using fastient.com. It's a website with similar features to the apps and great for someone looking for a site to track their progress. You can see an estimate on how many calories you've burnt in a fasting state and log your weight to see your results. Keep in mind that the calories burnt feature isn't entirely reliable but a rough estimate, but maybe it's motivating for you to see.

Technology has paved the ways of fasting and tracking the progress of fasting seems a lot easier with these technology buds.

5.4. Intermittent Fasting and Emotional Eating

Emotional eating or stress eating is the reason why so many diets fail. We don't always eat just to satisfy physical hunger. Many of us also use food to make ourselves feel better, eating to satisfy emotional needs, to relieve stress or cope with unpleasant emotions such as sadness, loneliness, or boredom. You might reach for a pint of ice cream when you're feeling down, order a pizza if you are bored or lonely, or feel better by the drive-through after a stressful day at work.

Occasionally using food as a pick-me-up, a reward, or to celebrate isn't necessarily a bad thing. But when eating is your primary emotional coping mechanism, when your first impulse is to open the refrigerator whenever you are stressed, upset, angry, lonely, exhausted, or bored. You get stuck in an unhealthy cycle where the real feeling or problem is never addressed. Emotional hunger can't be filled with food. Eating may feel good at the moment, but the feelings that triggered the eating are still there. You often feel worse than you did before because of the unnecessary calories you have just consumed.

Many people tend to incline towards emotional eating when they are under intense stress or emotions like boredom, sadness, and poor family relations. These people are known as emotional eaters. Emotional eaters strongly believe that eating is the answer to all their problems and food is a great stress reliever. It gives them the energy that they need. The point of caution is that too much of dependence on food is not very healthy.

Most emotional eaters eat food as a comfort measure and their dependence is often not detected until very late. Females are more emotional eaters than men are. Women tend to lean more towards salty, high calorie, sweet and fatty foods. These types of foods are not healthy and should be eaten in moderate portions. Emotional eaters especially women overindulge in these unhealthy foods. The most paradoxical part is that these comfort foods often make the eaters feeling guilty after the binge.

Various studies and research indicated a strong connection between stress and emotional eating which can be linked with brain chemistry. The fight or flight response in case of stress is also known to suppress the appetite. Nevertheless, in some cases of continuous stress people tend to turn towards comfort food for relief. The ironic part is that this type of food only adds to weight gain rather than reduce your stress.

You can avoid going on eating binges. The most important thing is to learn the difference between real hunger and emotional hunger. It is also helpful if you can identify and avoid food that activates emotional hunger in you.

Emotional eating can be very dangerous for your health and should be avoided at any cost. Too much of comfort foods can increase the risk of obesity and other diseases. Not to mention the social discomfort behind it. Right amount of exercise and a proper and correct diet can help you to avoid overeating. Exercise is also a great way to keep busy so that you do not feel stressed out. Regular lifestyle and exercise will help you in maintaining ideal weight and stop overeating.

No matter how powerless you feel over food and your feelings, it is possible to make a positive change. You can find healthier ways to deal with your emotions, learn to eat mindfully instead of mindlessly, regain control of your weight, and finally put a stop to emotional eating. Emotional hunger can be powerful, so it is easy to mistake it for physical hunger. But there are clues you can look for to help you tell physical and emotional hunger apart.

- Emotional hunger comes on suddenly. It hits you in an instant and feels overwhelming and urgent. Physical hunger, on the other hand, comes on more gradually. The urge to eat doesn't feel as dire or demand instant satisfaction (unless you haven't eaten for a very long time).
- Emotional hunger craves specific comfort foods. When you're physically hungry, almost anything sounds good—including healthy stuff like vegetables. But emotional hunger craves junk food or sugary snacks that provide an instant rush. You feel like you need cheesecake or pizza, and nothing else will do.
- Emotional hunger often leads to mindless eating. Before you know it, you've eaten a whole bag of chips or an entire pint of ice cream without really paying attention or fully

enjoying it. When you're eating in response to physical hunger, you're typically more aware of what you're doing.

- o Emotional hunger isn't satisfied once you're full. You keep wanting more and more, often eating until you're uncomfortably stuffed. Physical hunger, on the other hand, doesn't need to be stuffed. You feel satisfied when your stomach is full.

- o Emotional hunger isn't located in the stomach. Rather than a growling belly or a pang in your stomach, you feel your hunger as a craving you can't get out of your head. You're focused on specific textures, tastes, and smells.

- o Emotional hunger often leads to regret, guilt, or shame. When you eat to satisfy physical hunger, you're unlikely to feel guilty or ashamed because you're simply giving your body what it needs. If you feel guilty after you eat, it's likely because you know deep down that you're not eating for nutritional reasons.

This disrupts all the progress you have made until then with intermittent fasting. Therefore, it must be tackled with iron hands and proper strategies to eradicate and write it off.

5.5 How to stop emotional eating

Emotional hunger isn't easily quelled by eating. While filling up my work at the moment, eating because of negative emotions often leaves people feeling more upset than before? This cycle typically doesn't end until a person addresses emotional needs head-on.

- o   Find other ways to cope with stress

Discovering another way to deal with negative emotions is often the first step toward overcoming emotional eating. This could mean writing in a journal, reading a book, or finding a few minutes to otherwise relax and decompress from the day. It takes time to shift your mindset from reaching for food to engaging in other forms of stress relief, so experiment with a variety of activities to find what works for you.

- o   Move your body

Some people find relief in getting regular exercise. A walk or jog around the block or a quickie yoga routine may help in particularly emotional moments. In a research study, participants were asked to engage in eight weeks of yoga. They were then assessed on their mindfulness and insightful understanding. Basically their understanding of themselves and of situations surrounding them. The results showed that regular yoga may be a useful preventative measure to help diffuse emotional states such as anxiety and depression.

- o Try meditation

Others are calmed by turning inward to practices like meditation. There are a variety of studies that support mindfulness meditation as a treatment for binge eating disorder and emotional eating.

Simple deep breathing is a meditation that you can do almost anywhere. Sit in a quiet space and focus on your breath, slowly flowing in and out of your nostrils. You can browse sites like YouTube for free guided meditations. For example, Jason Stephenson's "Guided Meditation for Anxiety & Stress" has over 4 million views and goes through a series of visualization and breathing exercises for more than 30 minutes.

- ○ Start a food diary

Keeping a log of what you eat and when you eat it may help you identify triggers that lead to emotional eating. You can jot down notes in a notebook or turn to technology with an app like MyFitnessPal. While it can be challenging, try to include everything you eat, however big or small, and record the emotions you are feeling at that moment. Also, if you choose to seek medical help with your eating habits, your food diary can be a useful tool to share with your doctor.

- ○ Eat a healthy diet

Making sure you get enough nutrients to fuel your body is also key. It can be difficult to distinguish between true and emotional hunger. If you eat well throughout the day, it may be easier to spot when you're eating out of boredom or sadness or stress. Still facing the trouble? Try reaching for healthy snacks, like fresh fruit or vegetables, plain popcorn, and other low-fat, low-calorie foods.

- ○ Take common offenders out of your pantry

Consider trashing or donating foods in your cupboards that you often reach for in moments of strife. Think high-fat, sweet or calorie-laden things, like chips, chocolate, and ice cream. Also, postpone trips to the grocery store when you're feeling upset. Keeping the foods you crave out of reach when you are feeling emotional may help break the cycle by giving you time to think before noshing.

- o Pay attention to volume

Resist grabbing a whole bag of chips or other food to snack on. Measuring out portions and choosing small plates to help with portion control are mindful eating habits to work on developing.

Once you have finished one help, give yourself time before going back for a second. You may even want to try another stress-relieving technique, like deep breathing, in the meantime.

- o Seek support

Resist isolation in moments of sadness or anxiety. Even a quick phone call to a friend or family member can do wonders for your mood. There are also formal support groups that can help. Overeaters Anonymous is an organization that addresses overeating from emotional eating, compulsive overeating, and other eating disorders. Your doctor may give you a referral to a counselor or coach who can help you identify the emotions at the route of your hunger. Find other groups in your area by searching on social sites like Meetup.

- o Banish distractions

You may find yourself eating in front of the television, computer, or some other distraction. Try switching off the tube or putting down your phone the next time you find yourself in this pattern.

By focusing on your food, the bites you take, and your level of hunger, you may discover that you're eating emotionally. Some even find it helpful to focus on chewing 10 to 30 times before swallowing a bite of food. Doing these things gives your mind time to catch up to your stomach.

- o Work on positive self-talk

Feelings of shame and guilt are associated with emotional eating. It's important to work on the self-talk you experience after an episode, or it may lead to a cycle of emotional eating behavior.

Instead of coming down hard, try learning from your setback. Use it as an opportunity to plan for the future. And be sure to reward yourself with self-care measures, taking a bath, going for a leisurely walk, and so on. Overcoming emotional eating tends to involve teaching the sufferer healthier ways to view food and develop better eating habits, recognize their triggers for engaging in this behavior, and develop appropriate ways to prevent and alleviate stress. An important step in managing stress is exercise, since regular physical activity tends to dampen the production of stress chemicals, even leading to a decrease in depression, anxiety, and insomnia in addition to decreasing the tendency to engage in emotional eating.

Engaging in meditation and other relaxation techniques is also a powerful way to manage stress and therefore decrease emotional eating. Therefore, engaging in one or two meditation sessions a day can have lasting beneficial effects on health, even decreasing high blood pressure and heart rate.

Refraining from drug use and consuming no more than moderate amounts of alcohol are other important ways to successfully manage stress since many of these substances heighten the body's response to stress. Also, indulging in use of those substances often prevents the person from facing their problems directly so they are not able to develop effective ways to cope with or eliminate the stress.

Other lifestyle changes that can decrease stress include taking breaks at home and at work. Refrain from over-scheduling yourself. Learn to recognize and respond to your stress triggers. Take regular days off at intervals that are right for you. Structure your life to achieve a comfortable way to respond to the unexpected. For those who may need help dealing with stress, stress-management counseling in the form of individual or group therapy can be very useful. Stress counseling and group therapy have proven to reduce stress symptoms and improve overall health.

5.6. The maintenance phase

Five stages are identified for any type of behavioral or physical maintenance/change. The model was basically developed back in the 1970s. It has since been adapted for physical activity so that people incorporating healthy exercise can track their progress toward becoming regular exercisers. By knowing the stages, it is easier to foresee obstacles, stay focused and develop motivational techniques. These phases include:

- Pre-contemplation or Doing Nothing phase

Pre-contemplation is the stage of doing nothing. You may feel comfortable with your level of physical activity or lack thereof according to ACE Fitness. If someone else mentions a need for increased activity, you may deny it outright or ignore the advice. Even if presented with the dangers of inactivity, such as a greater risk for developing chronic conditions or diseases. A person in the pre-contemplation stage fluffs it off as happening someday or to someone else. Changing from pre-contemplation may require motivation that fosters confidence.

- Contemplation or Awareness Phase

Contemplation is the stage of awareness. Some people begin to notice they lose their breath more easily or their clothes no longer fit. This may be the stage of "I should . . ." statements, like "I should begin exercising," or "I should lose weight." It helps to set specific and target-oriented goals at this stage. Identify ways that change benefits you in order to motivate you to fulfill your goals.

- o Preparation or Planning Phase

Preparation is the planning stage when you decide how you will fulfill your goals. You may begin to use "I could . . ." statements, like "I could join a gym," or "I could run outside." At this stage, rely on experts for guidance or motivation to keep your plans realistic and attainable. As you progress from this stage, expect to feel a sense of mental readiness to enact your physical fitness goals.

- o The Hardest: Action phase

Action may be the hardest part of the five stages for many people. It's time to start working out. The Physical Activity Guidelines for Americans recommends getting at least 150 minutes of moderately-intense cardio exercise every week. That can translate to 30 minutes of activity per day for five days each week. You may perform all of this activity in one half-hour, or you may break it up into two 15-minute stretches. That can be daunting to someone who is just getting into a fitness routine. According to Rural Health Information Hub, the stages of change are cyclical and a person can easily slip from one stage back to another. If you feel a relapse into a prior stage is imminent, stay motivated with friends, trainers, regular weigh-ins, scheduled measurements or other quantitative reinforcements.

o   Phase of Accomplishment

The maintenance phase is a stage of accomplishment. Your clothes may fit differently. You may have a lower resting heart rate or perform more quickly for longer periods of time without needing rest. The danger now is that you'll rest on your laurels and stop working out.

Setting aside all this, this maintenance phase could contribute to making your body recover if it has got weaken in intermittent fasting together with physical feasibilities. Maintenance is a long-term commitment. You can change your workout to stay motivated, but you have to keep working out. Your life has changed successfully from when you were in the first stages of change.

Now let's talk about weight-maintenance phases, there are 3 main phases to maintain weight over the course of time. These are discussed below in detail:

❖ The Pre-Diet Weight-Maintenance phase

What It Is: The pre-diet weight-maintenance phase can be described as a four to the twelve-week period before a diet in which you focus on developing and consistently implementing healthy and sustainable eating habits.

Major Benefit: By developing these skills prior to a dieting phase, you will significantly increase the likelihood of success during your diet. Importantly, you will also master the ability to eat healthily and confidently for life, which significantly reduces the likelihood of regaining the weight you lost after your diet is over.

Remember that a dieting phase is a major physical and psychological stress. Trying to develop and sustain new skills during this time assuming you haven't spent time developing them prior) will only make this period more challenging—and will make healthy habits less likely to stick. But by spending time focusing on these new eating habits without the stress of a calorie deficit, you're far more likely to become proficient in them.

Optimal Duration: This phase should last four to twelve weeks. However, you should not proceed with a diet until you feel comfortable in your eating habits and consistency!

Note: This phase is especially important if you have a history of yo-yo or chronic dieting, or if you frequently catch yourself falling back on old eating habits. It's not a glamorous phase, and we know you'd rather jump right into a diet, but the benefit it provides in the long-term when implemented correctly is truly priceless.

❖ The post-diet weight-maintenance phase

What It Is: The post-diet weight-maintenance phase can be described as a three to the six-month period after a successful diet. During this phase, you make a series of gradual increases in your baseline calorie intake. The reason? To restore the physiological and psychological changes that took place during your diet.

Major Benefit: A well-executed post-diet weight-maintenance phase will enable you to restore the many physiological and psychological changes that took place during your diet. Specifically, it will rev up your metabolism, reduce appetite-stimulating hormones, increase appetite-suppressing hormones, and increase thyroid hormone production. Additionally, this phase serves as a psychological and physical reprieve from the stress of dieting.

At the end of this phase, when done correctly, you will be eating nearly as many calories per day as you were when you started your diet, but have maintained your weight loss within a few pounds…

Note: This phase is essential for everyone. You need to gradually bring your calories back up so you're well-fueled and not ravenous around the clock. You want to be able to enjoy life, after all! This phase is especially important if you wish to diet again in the future, it will put you in the best position possible to achieve successful weight loss during that time.

❖ The Forever Weight-Maintenance Phase

What It Is: The forever weight-maintenance phase can be described as the phase you are ultimately seeking! It's pure bliss, an everlasting phase in which you're confident in the way you look and feel, as well as how your clothes fit and how you're performing in the gym.

Major Benefit: This phase is like cruise control: you've achieved your desired look, feel, and performance and now want to maintain it while still making gradual improvements across the board. You're so pleased with everything that dieting is not on your mind or in your long-term plan for the foreseeable future or ever again.

At this stage in your nutrition journey, you've gone through the numerous ups and downs that come with losing weight and trying to maintain it. You're proficient in handling these challenges and are un-phased by small changes in weight, social occasions, and more.

How Long Should This Phase Last: Your forever weight maintenance phase can last, well, forever!

You may have spent the last year or longer achieving the weight, look, and feel you desired, and have spent even longer maintaining this weight.

CONCLUSION

Talking about the climax of this book, intermittent fasting drives and produces opportunities for the persons involving in its scenario the basic and comprehensive belongings of reshaping their bodies, building their muscles, and letting them find a viable way to maintain and build their body for a long period of time.

This has been done through various activates and pre-cautions to rest and acknowledge these efforts. Standard methods are developed for intermittent fasting that involves 16:8 method, eat-stop-eat method and 5:2 methods to simply put someone who is willing to join, in a marvelous way of reshaping their bodies, ad building their physique. These methods tried and tested with various expert's suggestions and opinions. If one adopts these methods, he/she must do some homework before adopting. As he/she has to assess his/her body conditions, know the values and requirements of the concerning method and let his body settle down with various implementations.

These methods cater to various benefits that allow the body to settle and turn into a comprehensive favorable situation that is required such as weight loss, which is the primary goal behind adopting these methods. This is accomplished with proper fat burning and preventing fat accumulation in the body, resulting in long-run fat avoidance.

Necessary pre-cautions or pre-requisites include the determination, courage and feel enthusiastic while adopting and maintaining intermittent fasting method. One must stick to his plan, try only prescribed conditions of food, exercise, and tryouts. This will result in the benefits and gets that are demanded and expected. The only condition is courage and determination!

Made in the USA
San Bernardino,
CA